Get fit for the Games

First published by Carlton Books Limited 2010
Copyright © 2010 Carlton Books Limited

London 2012 emblem(s)™ © The London Organising Committee
of the Olympic Games and Paralympic Games Ltd (LOCOG) 2007.
All rights reserved.

Carlton Books Limited
20 Mortimer Street
London W1T 3JW

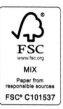
A CIP catalogue record for this book is available from the British Library.
10 9 8 7 6 5 4 3 2 1

ISBN: 978-1-84732-725-3

Editor: Matt Lowing
Design Direction: Darren Jordan
Designer: Ben Ruocco
Picture Research: Paul Langan
Production: Karin Kolbe
Photography: Karl Adamson
Editorial: Richard Gilbert, Lesley Levene, Lara Maiklem and Helen Whitton

Peta Bee is an award-winning journalist with degrees in sports science
and in nutrition. She currently writes a weekly fitness column in *The
Times* and is contributing editor of *Women's Running* magazine. In her
youth, Peta competed internationally at athletics and now coaches a
group of runners in her area. She has appeared widely on television
and radio and is the author of four previous books on health and fitness.
In 2003 Peta was voted Fitness Professional of the Year and she won the
Medical Journalists' Association's Freelance of the Year award in 2008.

Get fit for the Games

Every woman's total fitness workout

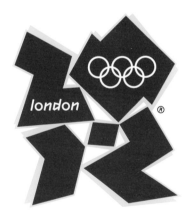

london

Peta Bee

CARLTON

Contents

Foreword by
Victoria Pendleton MBE

Winning the gold medal at the Beijing 2008 Olympic Games was one of the greatest moments of my life and I will cherish the memory forever.

I have loved all sports for as long as I can remember. Cycling, in particular, has been an important part of my life since I was very young and it has been a great source of happiness and fun for me, to say nothing of the joy of winning big events. With the London 2012 Olympic and Paralympic Games taking place on home soil, it will be even more exciting. It is the greatest sporting event ever held in the country and I can't wait for it to start.

The aim of this book is to make you feel part of the Games and inspire everyone to get in shape ready for when the London 2012 Games begin. It is never too late to start getting fit and no matter what your current fitness level may be, with some hard work – it is never easy – and determination, you will quickly discover the benefits that regular exercise and training can bring. At the end of this book, you may not get to step on the podium, but you will certainly feel better about yourself, and that is half the battle.

Victoria Pendleton MBE

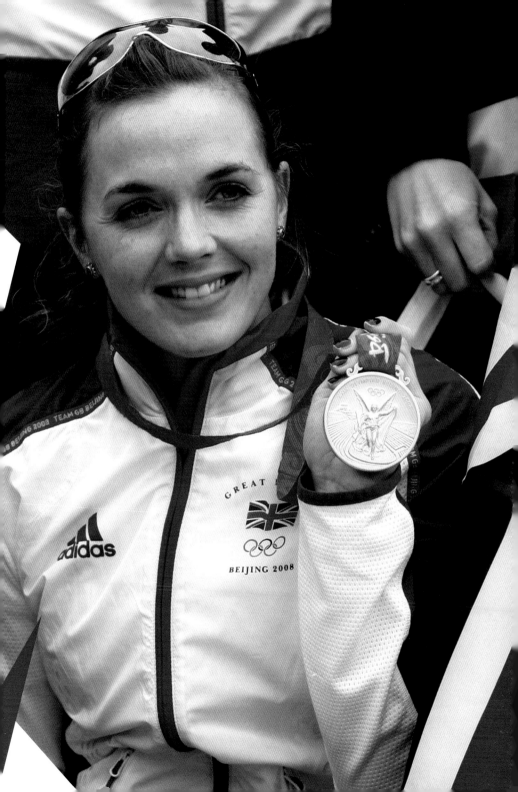

Introduction

Welcome to *Get fit for the Games*, the official women's fitness book of the London 2012 Olympic Games and Paralympic Games. If you are seeking inspiration and guidance to take your fitness to a new level, then you have selected the right book. This is not a guide to becoming an Olympic champion. Rather, its pages promise to steer you to a new level of personal achievement and glory. It is hoped the prospect of the Olympic Flame burning brightly in London in 2012 will ignite ambition in everyone to become fitter, stronger and healthier.

While the London 2012 Games will be a celebration of the cream of the world's athletes at the pinnacle of their careers, it is hoped its legacy is that it will be remembered as everyone's Games. It was Baron Pierre de Coubertin, the founder of the modern Olympics, who underlined the spirit of the movement when he declared, 'the most important thing in the Olympic Games is not winning but taking part; the essential thing in life is not conquering but fighting well.' That motto remains as relevant today as it always has been, with its meaning extended this time around to include anyone inspired to take part in sport or physical activity as a result of the London 2012 Games.

Each of the exercise programmes in this book is based on conditioning and strengthening moves used by top athletes looking to improve their basic fitness in a range of sports. They are as relevant to you as they are to an Olympic champion and have been modified and formulated into workouts designed to suit everyone from complete beginners to more experienced exercisers. Olympic athletes thrive on variety and new challenges to the training

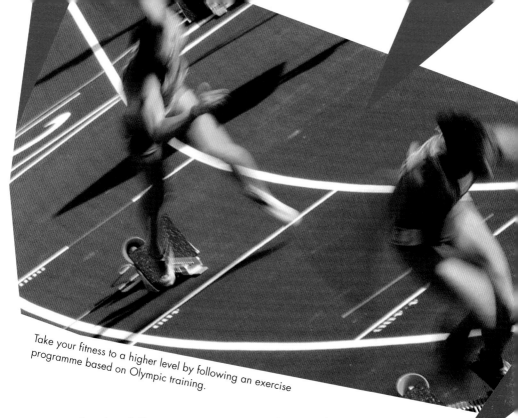

Take your fitness to a higher level by following an exercise programme based on Olympic training.

regimes that they follow in pursuit of their dreams. Like the rest of us, they get bored, stale and lack motivation if their workouts become too mundane or too complicated. Getting fit is as much about addressing the needs of the mind as those of the body. That is reflected in the way the Bronze, Silver and Gold workouts offer scope for change and progression without taking you out of your depth. Let the Games inspire you. Aim higher than you have done before and discover how well your own body can perform.

'We have always been clear — we want London 2012 to be everyone's Games and inspiring change through the 2012 Olympic Games and Paralympic Games was a cornerstone of our bid.'

Seb Coe, Chair of the London Organising Committee of the Olympic Games and Paralympic Games.

How to use this book

Get fit for the Games is designed to be a manual that offers advice, tips and guidelines to help you reach your fitness goals whatever your starting point. It is structured so that you can dip into and out of its pages to gain specific information whenever you need.

There are three main sections to the book – the Basics, the Workouts and the Practicalities. In the first section, you are introduced to the different elements of fitness and how they apply to your body. There's advice on what to wear and what equipment you need to get started. Also explained is the importance of warming up and cooling down.

The second section contains details of the exercises involved in the three 12-week workouts. These are progressive, which means your fitness levels will continue to improve as advance

Fitness is not all about exercising and the third section addresses the practicalities of an active lifestyle. It includes tips on staying motivated and a troubleshooting guide to common niggles and complaints.

Safety notes

Before you embark on the workout programmes, complete the safety questionnaire on page 11 and the series of assessments that begins on page 30. They will give you a better idea of your current fitness level and help to make sure that you begin with the workout that is most appropriate.

Always make sure that you are wearing appropriate clothing and that the room where you will be working out is well-ventilated and adequately spacious. Remove any objects that could be knocked over or broken and make sure the floor surface is not wet or slippery. Have water to hand in case you get dehydrated and check that any equipment is in working order.

Getting started safely

Starting an exercise programme is considered the best step most people can take to improve their health and well-being. But before you get going, there are a number of questions to ask yourself to make sure it is safe for you to start.

If you haven't exercised for a while or have any underlying health problems it is wise to make an appointment to see your GP for a health check. If you are aged 70 or over it is also advisable to seek your doctor's advice before starting to exercise. Answer the questions below:

• Do you have a history of heart disease in your family or have you ever been told you have a heart problem?
• Do you ever feel pain or tightness in your chest muscles when you are being active?
• Have you been told you have high blood pressure (i.e. above 160/90)?
• Do you ever feel dizzy or faint or do you ever lose consciousness?
• Do you have old injuries that cause you pain when you move?

• Do you suffer from chronic back pain?
• Do you have osteoporosis, arthritis or any other joint or bone problem that could deteriorate if you exercise?
• Are you overweight or obese (use the BMI or WHR tests on page 41 to check)?
• Are you pregnant?
• Are you taking any medication prescribed by your doctor?

If you answered 'yes' to one or more of the questions above, then book an appointment with your GP. They will give you a thorough health check and, with luck, the green light to embark on this programme. If you answered 'no' to each of the questions above, then your next step is to assess your fitness and get on the starting blocks to a new, fitter you.

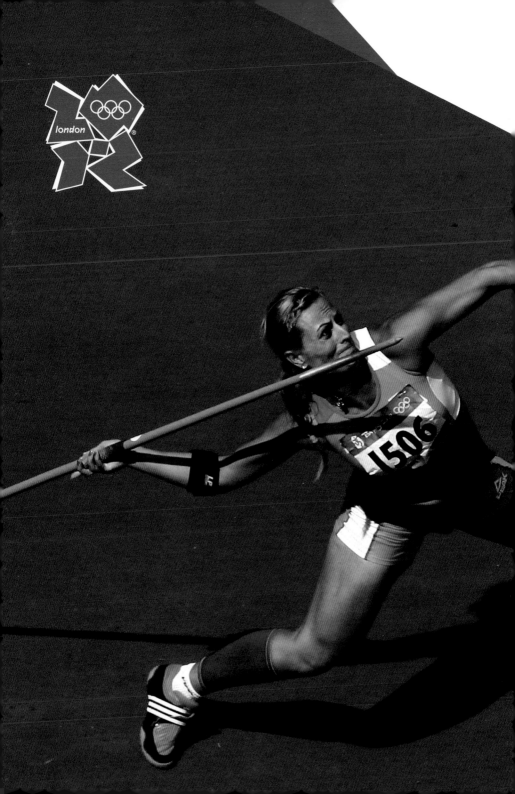

The basics

Olympic and Paralympic athletes devote their lives to training regimes that enable them to compete for medals. But fitness means many things to many people and, along with improved strength, endurance and flexibility, it can boost your self-esteem and even extend your life.

Each Olympic sport requires specific exercises, as well as general conditioning and strengthening moves, which can help anyone improve their basic fitness.

The basics – introduction

To watch Olympians or Paralympians compete at the pinnacle of their career is to marvel at their grace, speed, strength and powers of endurance. With bodies and minds so finely tuned to achieve peak performance, they are supreme examples of what the human body can achieve with talent, effort and dedication.

The fitness levels of a top athlete might seem a world away from what you are hoping to achieve from an exercise programme. But whether your goal is to run in an Olympic final or run around the block, the fundamental benefits of exercise and the basics of what is entailed when it comes to improving fitness are the same.

Before you embark on the road to a fitter, stronger self, it is crucial to have a basic understanding of where you are coming from and where you hope your exercise programme will lead. The human body is an amazing and complex structure comprising more than 200 bones, 650 voluntary muscles (those over which you have some control) and interchangeable energy systems designed to cope with all levels of physical activity.

This section of the book looks at how your body works and what it means to be fit. It addresses the steps you need to take to make sure you are ready to get started and introduces the warm-up, cool-down and stretching exercises that are the support system of all exercise programmes, minimising the risk of injury and enabling your body to move in the way Mother Nature intended.

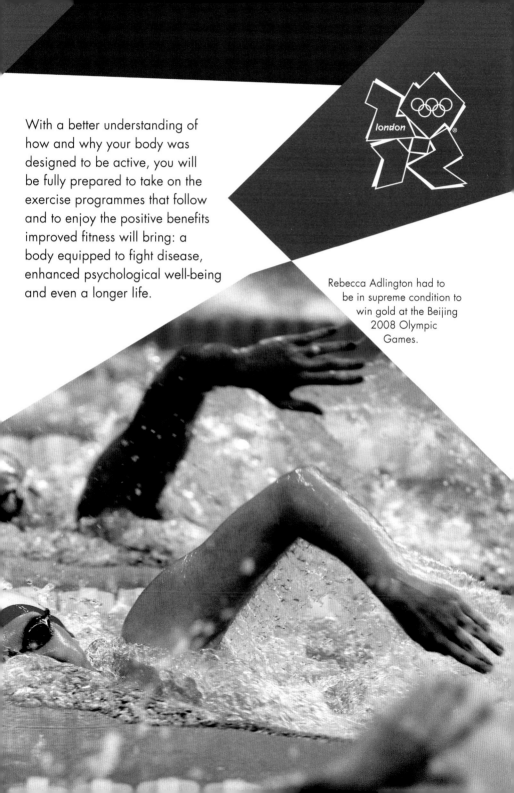

With a better understanding of how and why your body was designed to be active, you will be fully prepared to take on the exercise programmes that follow and to enjoy the positive benefits improved fitness will bring: a body equipped to fight disease, enhanced psychological well-being and even a longer life.

Rebecca Adlington had to be in supreme condition to win gold at the Beijing 2008 Olympic Games.

Aerobic fitness explained

Whatever their sport, athletes devote a significant part of training to improving their aerobic or cardiovascular fitness. During exercise, your muscles need to use more oxygen than they would if you were standing still. As the mainstay of any physical activity programme, aerobic fitness improves stamina by enabling your heart, lungs and blood vessels to deliver oxygen and nutrients to the working muscles more efficiently. The result? You can keep going for longer.

So how is aerobic fitness improved? Aerobic means 'with oxygen' and aerobic exercise tends to engage the body's largest muscles – such as those in the legs and arms – in movements that are sustained and repetitive. Distance running, swimming and cycling are all good examples, but you can also boost your aerobic capacity through simple everyday activities like skipping, walking and climbing stairs.

The key to forming a good aerobic base is to start gently. Begin with 2–3 weekly sessions of 20–30 minutes of aerobic activity at a pace and intensity you find comfortable. Try to move too quickly in the early stages and your body will struggle to supply the oxygen required. When this happens, the exercise becomes 'anaerobic' (meaning 'without oxygen'), your legs quickly feel heavy and tired and you are forced to stop prematurely.

Once your cardiovascular fitness improves, however, you can begin to increase the duration and variety of

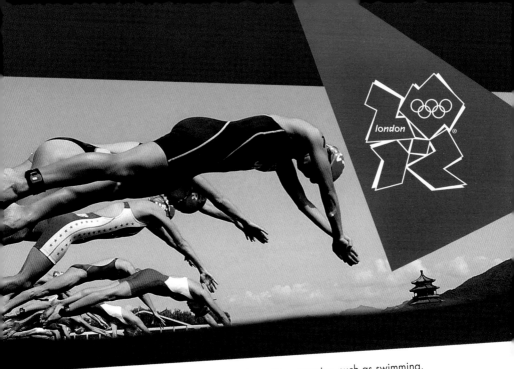

Aerobic fitness can be improved by sustained and repetitive exercise, such as swimming.

your workouts. Try to vary the intensity of your aerobic sessions as much as possible. Athletes combine bursts of speed with bouts of less effort to push themselves into more demanding training zones, but the same effect can be achieved by mixing walking with running or periods of gentle cycling with all-out effort.

Within weeks of becoming more aerobically active, you will find that your resting heart rate – the average number of heart beats per minute – will drop, a sign that your heart is pumping more powerfully and your lungs working more efficiently than

before. Sports physiologists have shown that aerobic exercise triggers the release of feel-good chemicals from the brain, called endorphins, that flood into the bloodstream and improve your mood. With your metabolism boosted, calories will be gobbled up at a faster rate. What reason is there not to get moving?

Olympic sports that provide the best aerobic workout	
Athletics – distance running	Cycling
	Boxing
Swimming	Water Polo
Rowing	Football

17

Strength fitness explained

A strong body is a healthy body. In many Olympic events, strength is crucial to performance as it is required, along with speed, to produce the power needed to jump, sprint or throw. You may not need to attain the levels of strength displayed by Olympians, but improving your body's overall strength will have a profound impact on your fitness levels, general health and appearance.

But how do you go about getting stronger? A common mistake is to assume that strength training can only be performed in the weights room or at the gym. In fact, muscles become stronger when presented with any force that provides weight or resistance – that includes household items like bottles filled with water or sand, cans of beans or tomatoes and gravity, in the form of your own body weight.

Muscles respond to weights or resistance by exerting a force, pulling on bones to maintain a particular position or help the body move in a particular way. The more often

muscles are overloaded in this way, the better they adapt to the demands and the stronger they eventually become. Strength fitness sections, such as those in this book, are usually structured according to the number of repetitions (or reps) of a particular exercise that are required, the number of sets (groups of repetitions performed in succession) and the amount of rest you will need to take in between.

How many repetitions you perform and how heavy the weights or strong the resistance you use depend on the type of strength improvements you are trying to achieve. Higher

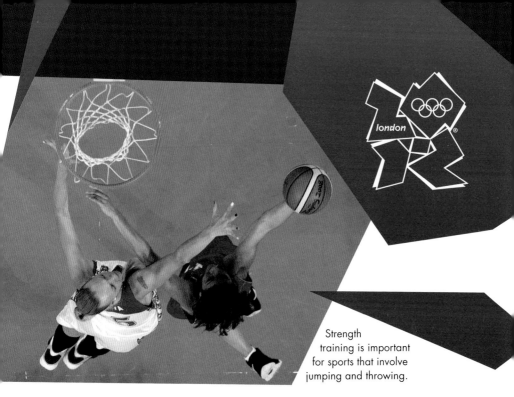

Strength training is important for sports that involve jumping and throwing.

repetitions of lower weights are lifted to improve muscular endurance, the kind of strength needed to perform everyday activities and to improve general fitness. Athletes looking to improve pure muscular strength, the kind needed in power and strength-based sports, will lift heavy weights just a couple of times.

There's little doubt that strength fitness will pay dividends. Stronger muscles mean more lean muscle mass and less fatty tissue; metabolically active muscle tissue burns calories at a faster rate, so if weight loss is your aim, you will reach the goal more quickly. Resistance training is known to strengthen bones, protecting against the bone-thinning disease osteoporosis, and some researchers have shown that women who lift weights have a better body image than those who don't. And, in case you are in doubt, women who weight train rarely add bulk. Instead they end up with supremely toned and lean bodies.

Olympic sports that rely on strength and power	
Weightlifting	Boxing
Gymnastics	Diving
Athletics – throwing events	Judo
	Athletics –
Wrestling	jumping events

Stretching and flexibility explained

Watch young children play and you'll see they are naturally flexible, their bodies moving in the way they were designed to by reaching and stretching in different directions and planes. From childhood onwards that range of movement diminishes as age, our lifestyles and general wear and tear, plus postural bad habits, take their toll, causing muscles and tendons around the joints to shorten and joints to stiffen, reducing functional range.

It is precisely to prevent such a decline that flexibility and stretching programmes are a key component of any Olympic athlete's training. Intense physical activity causes muscle fibres to contract and shorten, which can be detrimental to performance unless redressed. With regular stretching, the muscles and tendons are lengthened again, leading to greater flexibility and a body that moves freely through a wide range of motion.

Indeed, athletes skimp on stretching and flexibility at their peril. An inflexible body is more prone to injury. Not only are stiff muscles and joints vulnerable to sprains and strains when sudden movements are made, but muscular imbalances can occur when restricted flexibility affects one or more parts of the body. Someone who spends hours driving or hunched over a computer keyboard, for instance, will compensate for the lack of movement and flexibility in some muscles by stressing others.

Regular stretching has other benefits. It improves the flow of blood to

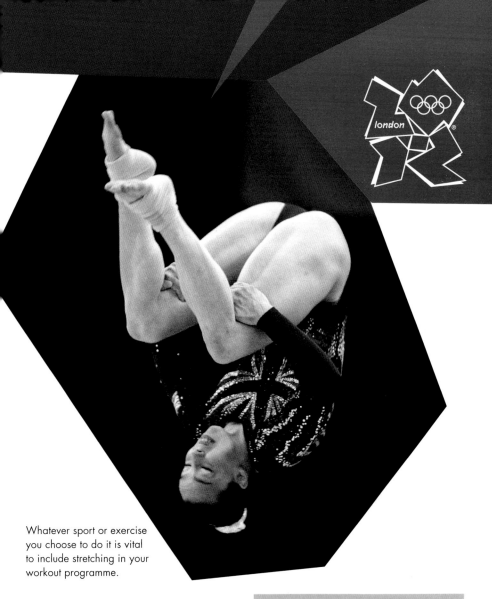

Whatever sport or exercise you choose to do it is vital to include stretching in your workout programme.

joints, helping to keep them fluid and mobile, and can also be a time to help body and mind relax and unwind. Whatever your sport or fitness goals, total-body stretching for all-round flexibility is essential if you want to achieve them.

Olympic sports that rely on stretching and flexibility

Gymnastics	**Athletics –**
Athletics –	**jumping events**
throwing events	**Diving**
Judo	**Modern Pentathlon**

Muscle identification — front of the body

If you understand where the major muscle groups are positioned it will help you 'feel' if an exercise is working the right areas.

Biceps: Positioned at the front of the upper arm. Used to bend the arm at the elbow.

Deltoids: A group of muscles in the shoulder area that are used in lifting, pulling and other powerful movements involving the arms.

Pectorals (pecs): Span the chest area and are used to move the arm across the body as well as in pushing movements.

Rectus abdominus (abs): Sometimes known as the six-pack muscle, it is the long, flat muscle that extends vertically between the pubic bone and the fifth, sixth and seventh ribs. It is used to help maintain posture and to bend the trunk forwards.

External abdominal obliques: Located on each side of the rectus abdominus and used to flex and rotate the trunk.

Internal abdominal obliques: Lie under the external oblique muscle and are engaged when flexing the trunk to the same side as the muscle.

Transversus abdominus: The deepest layer of abdominal muscle, it wraps around the torso like a corset from front to back and from ribs to torso. It stabilises the spine and compresses the abdomen.

Hip flexors: A group of muscles that sit at the front of the hip and bring the legs and trunk together in a flexion movement.

Adductors: Often referred to as groin muscles, they are fan-like muscles in the upper thigh that are used to pull the leg inwards.

Quadriceps (quads): A group of four muscles located in the front of the thigh. Used to extend the leg while straightening the knee in running and jumping.

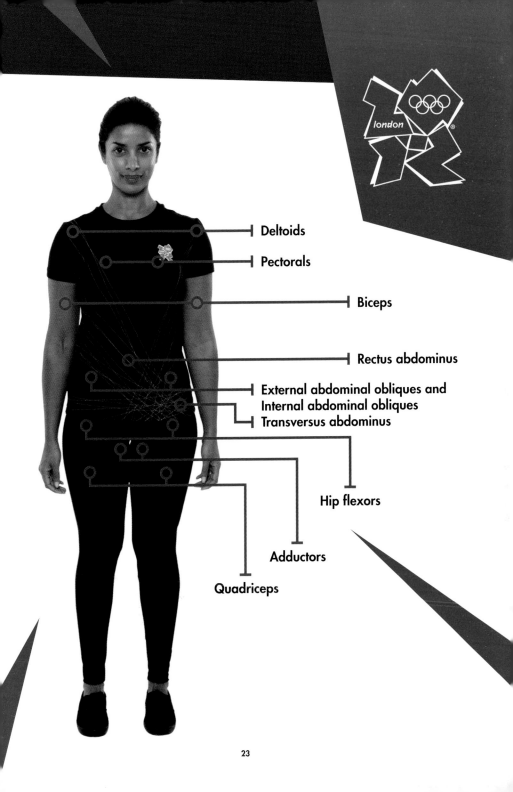

Deltoids

Pectorals

Biceps

Rectus abdominus

External abdominal obliques and
Internal abdominal obliques
Transversus abdominus

Hip flexors

Adductors

Quadriceps

Muscle identification – back of the body

Rhomboids: Positioned in the middle of the back between the shoulder blades. Used to protect the spine and to draw the arms and shoulders backwards in movements like rowing.

Trapezius: A large, triangular muscle on either side of the upper back, extending from the shoulder to the neck. Used to move the shoulder blades upwards in actions such as shrugging.

Latissimus dorsi (lats): A broad, triangular, flat muscle that spans your back and is connected to bones in your spine, shoulder and arms. Used to lower the arms towards the body.

Triceps: Positioned in the back of the upper arm and used to straighten the arm out at the elbow.

Quadratus lumborum: Located at the sides and slightly to the back of the waist. Used for side-bending movements and to stabilise the spine and pelvis.

Erector spinae: A group of three muscles that span the length of the spine, running along the neck to the lower back. Used to protect, lengthen and stabilise the spine, as well as in backwards movement.

Multifidus: Located beneath the erector spinae and runs along the sides of the spinal column. Used to extend and rotate the spine.

Gluteus maximus (glutes): Located in the buttocks. Used to pull the leg back or push the body upwards.

Hip abductors: The gluteus medius and gluteus minimus muscles located on the hips form the hip abductor muscles. They are used to lift the leg sideways away from the body.

Hamstrings: Located at the back of the upper leg. Used to bend the knee and extend the hip.

Calf muscles: The gastrocnemius is the big calf muscle at the back of the lower leg and the soleus the smaller muscle beneath it. Together they work to push the foot down and stabilise the legs' position during running and walking.

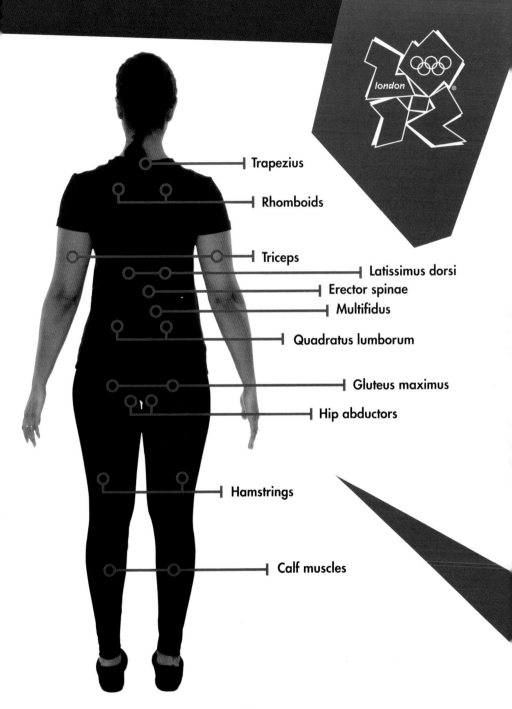

Trapezius

Rhomboids

Triceps

Latissimus dorsi

Erector spinae

Multifidus

Quadratus lumborum

Gluteus maximus

Hip abductors

Hamstrings

Calf muscles

Clothing

A workout wardrobe can be as extensive or minimal as you choose. It is not necessary to spend a fortune on chic and stylish gym wear (although some people adhere to the adage that if you look good, then you will feel good), but investing in some fitness clothing staples will certainly help you to exercise in more comfort.

Sports bra: Among the most essential items of clothing for active women is a good sports bra. You don't need to be big-busted to need the support they provide and failure to wear one when performing any kind of repetitive or high-impact activity can take its toll in the long term. Irreversible sagging is a risk with unsupportive bras – the Cooper's ligaments, which act as a fragile support system for the breast tissue, get stretched to their limits. Over time this can also lead to back and shoulder pain. It is worth visiting a specialist shop to get measured – around 85 per cent of sporty women wear the wrong size of bra, which further reduces the support it provides.

Trainers: If you are going to splash out on an item of fitness clothing,

make it the footwear. Running shoes provide support for activities that involve linear or forward motion so are suitable for running, walking and performing most of the exercises in this book (although they can also be done barefoot). A good cross-trainer provides the kind of support needed in sports and activities (like aerobics classes) that involve changes in direction, twisting or turning. Specialist shoes are recommended if you do a lot of a particular sport, such as cycling, tennis or football. Whatever the trainers, always try them on in the afternoon when your feet are at their most swollen and take along your old pair so that the staff can look at the outer sole and insole to see where you land with most pressure. Generally they should be a size bigger than your

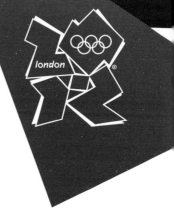

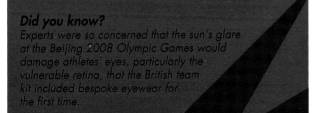
everyday shoes – there should be a 1 centimetre gap between the end of the longest toe and the shoe to allow for movement during exercise.

Sunglasses: Sunglasses are not just a fashion accessory. They protect your eyes against damaging rays and also enhance vision on sunny days – essential to achieve peak performance in some sports.

Hat: A peaked, baseball-style cap is great for keeping the sun's glare out of your eyes and protecting the top of your head from UV rays in the summer, while a warmer hat can help your body to maintain heat when you exercise outdoors in the winter.

Socks: They may seem an inconsequential item of fitness clothing

– unless you are prone to blisters when you exercise. If so, specialist seam-free sports socks, which often feature extra cushioning in the heel for added comfort, are a blessing.

Summer wear: For shorts, leggings and tops choose modern sweat-wicking fabrics with mesh panels to keep you cool. Steer clear of traditional cotton, which absorbs sweat rather than dispersing it.

Winter wear: Layering is the key to outdoor winter exercise. Lightweight, sweat-wicking tops are easy to peel off and keep you just as toasty as a thick fleece. A pair of lightweight gloves is useful if you suffer from cold hands and invest in a breathable waterproof jacket if you go running or walking outdoors.

Equipment

Minimal equipment is needed to carry out the workouts in this book. In fact, you can get by with just plastic bottles filled with water or sand as hand weights in the early stages of your fitness programme. However, the following might be useful:

Weights: There is a wide variety of weights and resistance-training accessories including everything from medicine balls to elastic resistance bands, but a set of dumbbells is a good starting point for any fitness programme. Choose either a set with different weighted dumbbells or one with removable discs that allow you to alter the weight as necessary.

Bench: Although you can manage without a workout bench for the exercises in this book, it is a worthwhile purchase if you have room to use and store it at home. If you purchase one, make sure it is sturdy enough to carry your weight and that it has an incline setting for varied exercises.

Exercise mat: Stretching is a vital aspect of the Get fit for the Games

programmes and a non-slip, slightly cushioned and washable exercise mat is a great (and cheap) investment if you are doing exercises at home on hard flooring.

Exercise step: This can be used for strength training and also to perform aerobic workouts. It is easily stored away. Choose one that is hard-wearing, offers different heights and is sturdy when you step onto it.

Pedometer: These devices range from basic models that simply tally the number of steps you have walked or run to high-tech versions that calculate the distance you cover and the calories you burn during exercise, with results that can be downloaded onto your computer. However, research published in the British Journal of Sports Medicine

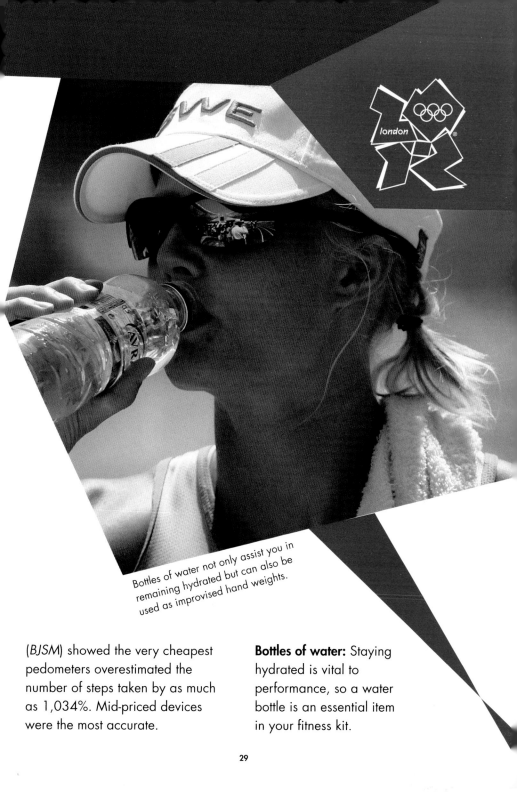

Bottles of water not only assist you in remaining hydrated but can also be used as improvised hand weights.

(*BJSM*) showed the very cheapest pedometers overestimated the number of steps taken by as much as 1,034%. Mid-priced devices were the most accurate.

Bottles of water: Staying hydrated is vital to performance, so a water bottle is an essential item in your fitness kit.

Assessing your fitness

Olympic athletes are constantly assessing and reassessing their fitness levels. The reason? They want to make sure that their training is heading in the right direction, that the hours they devote to the gym, track or pool are paying off. Regularly performing a range of physiological tests can give a clear idea of someone's state of fitness, as well as providing insight into aspects of training that may require more attention.

Your goals may not be Olympian in standard, but the principles of fitness testing remain the same: to provide you with a marker of your current fitness and to ensure that you start exercising at an appropriate level and intensity. On the pages that follow you will find eight exercises, each testing a particular aspect of your fitness, be it strength flexibility or endurance. Results of the tests will be used to direct you to the Bronze, Silver or Gold workouts later in the book.

After a thorough warm-up (see pages 48–55), perform each of the exercise tests, taking a 2–3 minute recovery break between each. Once you have completed the battery of tests, write down the results in a notebook or training diary. Repeat the entire fitness assessment every 6–8 weeks, always remembering to record your results. As you get stronger and fitter, your score in the tests should improve, providing a great source of motivation now the effort you are putting in is paying dividends. But fitness tests are also designed to reveal weaknesses and fitness vulnerabilities. If the results of your tests begin to drop off or plateau for several months on the trot, it may

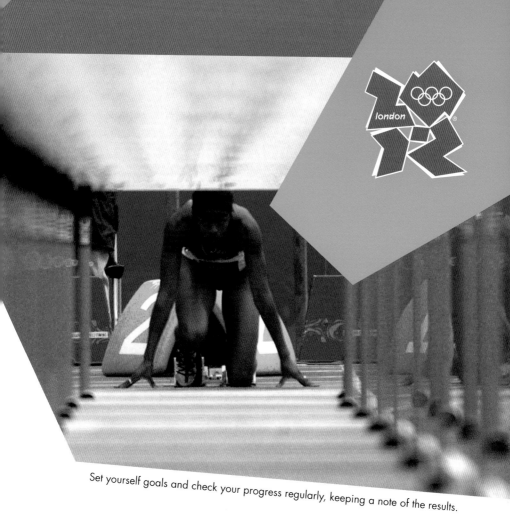

Set yourself goals and check your progress regularly, keeping a note of the results.

be time to look more closely at your lifestyle as a whole. It could be that you need to think about increasing the duration, intensity or frequency of your exercise to see improvements. Or that your lack of progress is being hampered by stresses in other areas of your life – an unusually heavy workload, a house move or career change. Put the results into

perspective and use them as a guide to propel you forward.

You will find some of the tests more demanding than others and should perform the entire assessment on a day when you have no other workout planned. Remember to use good technique and to cool down properly (see pages 58–61) when you finish.

Box press-up test

To assess:
Upper body strength and muscular endurance.

How to do the test:
Kneel on all fours with your knees hip-width apart and your arms directly beneath your shoulders, fingers facing forwards. Make sure your back is flat and your head in line with your spine.

Breathe in as you bend your elbows and lower your upper body towards the floor. Try to touch the floor with the tip of your nose. Hold that position briefly before pressing back up to the start position with your arms. Make sure the movement is fluid and repeat in fairly quick succession.

Results:
0–8 – Bronze
9–16 – Silver
17 plus – Gold

Did you know?
Drinking chocolate-flavoured milk – a favourite of American swimmer Michael Phelps, who has won 14 Olympic gold medals – after exercise could help stimulate muscle protein synthesis that boosts the recovery process, according to nutritionists at the American College of Sports Medicine.

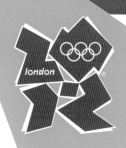

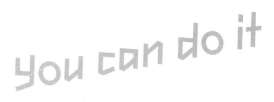

You can do it

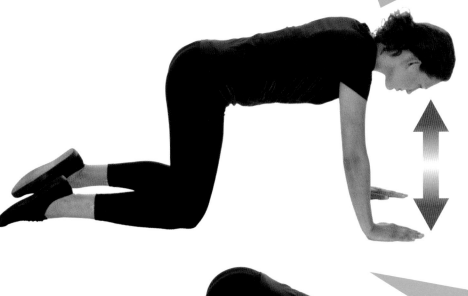

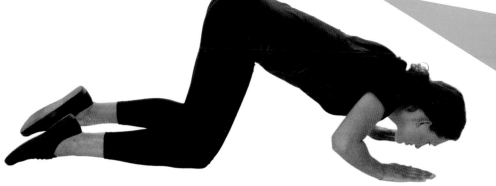

Abdominal hold

To assess:
Abdominal strength and muscular endurance in the trunk and hip flexor muscles.

How to do the test:
Sit on the floor with your back straight and knees bent with your feet flat on the floor. Stretch your arms out in front of you at shoulder height. Place your feet about hip-width apart and slowly lean back to the point where your hands are above your bent knees (but not touching them). Keep your back straight and head up, eyes looking forward. Hold the V-position for as long as you comfortably can. How long can you stay in position?

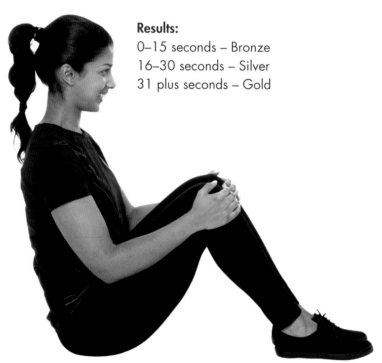

Results:
0–15 seconds – Bronze
16–30 seconds – Silver
31 plus seconds – Gold

Assessing your fitness

Hold it

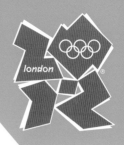

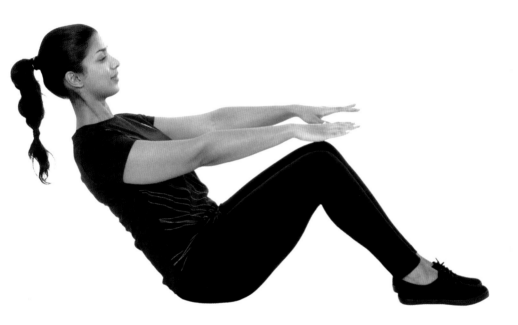

Did you know?
Gail Emms, who won a silver medal in badminton at the 2004 Olympic Games, spent up to an hour every day in the weights room building her strength and ran for at least 40 minutes 5–6 days a week, on top of the several hours a day of on-court drills and match play.

Chairless sit

To assess:
Strength and muscular endurance in the legs and lower body.

How to do the test:
Stand approximately 50cm away from a wall with your feet hip-width apart, hips square to the front and feet facing forward. Bend your knees and lower your back against the wall in a seated position but without the chair. There should be a 90-degree angle between hips and knees, so shuffle your feet forward if your knees are too far over your feet. Keep your shoulders relaxed and pressed into the wall. Hold the position for as long as you can. For how many seconds can you sit?

Results:
0–30 seconds – Bronze
31–45 seconds – Silver
46 plus seconds – Gold

Safety notes
• *Don't perform exercises on a slippery floor surface or on a rug/mat that might move when you step on it.*
• *Make sure that all equipment you are using (such as chairs) is stable and can bear your weight before you attempt the relevant exercise.*

Forward flexibility

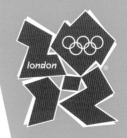

To assess:
Flexibility in the lower back.

How to do the test:
Sit with your back straight, hips facing forward and abdominal muscles tucked in. Position your legs in a V by extending them out to the sides. Slowly lean forward from your hips. Place lightly clenched fists on the floor, one on top of the other in the centre of the V created between your legs. Gradually lean your chest towards the top fist. How close can you get?

Results:
20cm plus from fists – Bronze
5cm–19cm from fists – Silver
Less than 5cm or touch fists – Gold

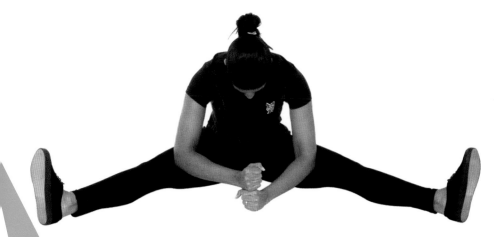

Sit and reach

To assess:
Flexibility in the hamstrings at the backs of the legs, hip flexors and lower back muscles.

How to do the test:
Sit on the floor with your legs extended in front of you and feet flexed. Make sure your back is straight and your abdominals are tucked in. Reach up towards the ceiling with your hands and then, bending from the hips, stretch your arms towards your toes. Try to keep your back flat and don't over-flex your neck muscles. How close do your fingertips come to your toes?

Results:
10cm plus from toes – Bronze
5–9cm from toes – Silver
Reach to or past toes – Gold

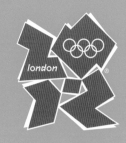

Did you know?
Britain's Olympic cycling gold medallist Nicole Cooke unwittingly began honing her fitness from the age of 11 when she would race her father twice daily on the 11-kilometre trip to and from secondary school.

Reach out

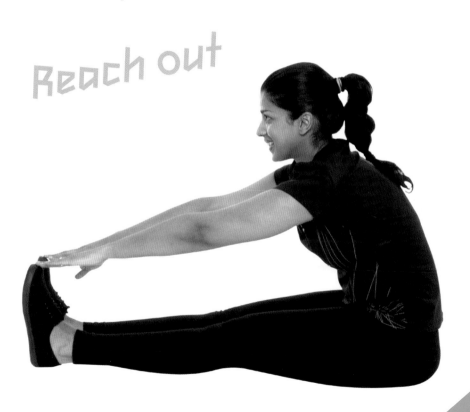

Training health checks

Athletes' bodies are like finely tuned machines that work well when they are in peak condition but need checking regularly to make sure they are functioning optimally. The kind of training health checks used by athletes are a useful guide for anyone embarking on a fitness programme. Carry out the following checks regularly, not only to assess your fitness but to see how well you are progressing with your activity programme.

Heart rate

Although it's a simple test, checking your pulse to find your heart rate remains one of the most widely used of all fitness tests, even among Olympic athletes. Your heart rate provides a straightforward means of ensuring your body is working at the right intensity during exercise. It can also help to determine when you are fully recovered from a bout of activity. Take your resting pulse rate first thing in the morning, when your body is at its most relaxed. All you need is a stopwatch or clock with a second hand.

Using the first two fingers of your right hand, feel for your pulse beneath the jawline on the muscle that runs down from your neck. When you have located your pulse, press down with the two fingers very gently. Counting 0 for the first beat, continue counting the number of beats in 15 seconds. Multiply by four to get the number of beats per minute. Make a record of your resting pulse rate and check it regularly. As you get fitter you should find the figure drops. A resting pulse rate of 70 or less is excellent. A good score is between 72 and 78. Checking your heart rate during exercise can help to make sure that you are working at the right intensity.

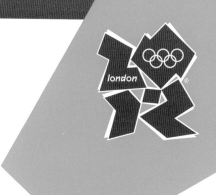

Body Mass Index (BMI)

Your BMI is an equation that has been widely used for many years to determine whether you are too heavy (or light) for your size. Since it doesn't take into account body composition – i.e. whether your weight comprises fat or muscle – it should be only used as a general guide, not a determinant of obesity. Beware that some muscular Olympians fall into the overweight category on the BMI scoring system. However, its appeal is its simplicity: your weight in kilograms is divided by your height in metres squared – the resulting figure being your BMI. For example:

Weight: 75kg
Height: 1.70m
Height squared (1.7 x 1.7) = 2.89
Weight divided by height squared (75 divided by 2.89) = 25.9

Your BMI result is then rated as follows:

A score below 18.5 = underweight
18.5–24.9 = a normal weight
25–29.9 = overweight
30 plus = clinically obese

Waist to Hip Ratio (WHR)

How heavy you are is not the only indicator of weight-related problems. What matters is how your body weight is distributed and this test helps to determine whether you are more prone to accumulating fat around the abdominal area (sometimes called an apple shape), which is considered less healthy than if you store weight on your hips (a pear shape). To work out your WHR score, measure your waist about 3cm above your navel to find your waist circumference and then measure your hips (just below the point where the top of the thigh bone meets the pelvis). Divide your waist circumference by your hip measurement to get your WHR. A ratio of below 0.85 is preferable and indicates that you store weight at the hips rather than the abdominal region.

Shoulder extension

To assess:
Flexibility in the triceps muscles in the backs of the arms and in the shoulders.

How to do the test:
Stand with your back straight and hips square to the front, feet hip-width apart. Bend your knees slightly and bend your left arm over your left shoulder, dropping the hand between the shoulder blades. Bend your right arm at the elbow and reach up behind your back to try and grab your left hand. How close together can you get your fingertips?

Results:
6cm plus between fingertips on one or both sides – Bronze
2cm plus between fingertips on one or both sides – Silver
You can grab hands on both sides – Gold

Feel great

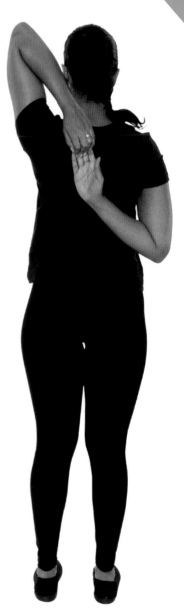

42

Crunch sit-up test

To assess:
Muscular strength and endurance in the abdominal region.

How to do the test:
Lie on your back with your knees bent and hip-width apart and feet flat on the floor. Press your lower back into the floor and contract your abdominal muscles tightly. Place both hands on the front of your thighs. Breathe in. As you exhale, slowly raise your shoulders off the floor in a small, controlled movement – the aim is not to lift them too far. Slide your palms up towards your knees, keeping your lower back down. Hold briefly at the top of the movement before lowering your shoulders back down. Keep your abdominal muscles contracted throughout. Allow your shoulders to brush the floor before repeating the move. Count how many you can do in a minute.

Results:
0–8 – Bronze
9–20 – Silver
21 plus – Gold

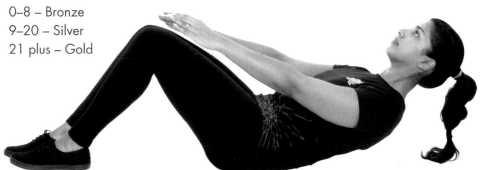

Step-up test

To assess:
Endurance.

How to do the test:
Stand facing a low-level bench or step, keeping your back straight and abdominal muscles contracted. Step up onto the bench with the whole of your left foot, then the whole of your right foot. Step back down, left foot first, then right foot. Breathe evenly throughout the exercise. Continue for 3 minutes. Sit down for 30 seconds before recording your pulse rate for 60 seconds (see page 40). What is the result?

Results:
50 bpm or greater above
your resting heart rate – Bronze
30–49 bpm above your
resting heart rate – Silver
29 or fewer bpm above your
resting heart rate – Gold

step up

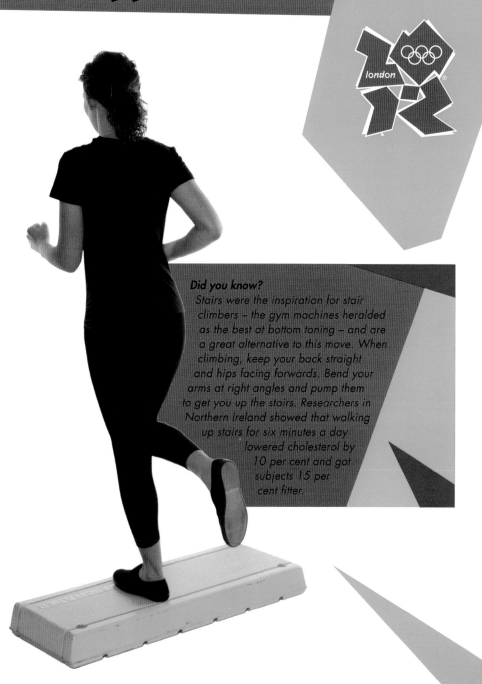

Did you know?
Stairs were the inspiration for stair climbers – the gym machines heralded as the best at bottom toning – and are a great alternative to this move. When climbing, keep your back straight and hips facing forwards. Bend your arms at right angles and pump them to get you up the stairs. Researchers in Northern Ireland showed that walking up stairs for six minutes a day lowered cholesterol by 10 per cent and got subjects 15 per cent fitter.

Assessing your fitness — summary

Now that you have completed the basic fitness assessment, it is time to find out the most appropriate *Get fit for the Games* programme for your current level. Remember that the assessments are intended as a guide only and it is also important to listen to your body and judge the way it responds to physical activity when deciding whether you are exercising at the right intensity. If you start a programme only to discover it is too easy or too hard, it is better to adjust your expectations and switch to an approach that better suits your needs than to plough on regardless.

Which workout is for you?
Try the Bronze workout if:
- You had four or more Bronze scores in the assessment.

- You are not very active and probably have not exercised (or exercised infrequently) for six months to a year.

Try the Silver workout if:
- You had four or more Silver scores in the assessment, but fewer than three Gold scores.

- You already lead an active lifestyle and probably do light to moderate exercise 2–3 times a week.

Try the Gold workout if:
- You had four or more Gold scores and fewer than three Bronze scores.

- You have been exercising consistently and regularly for a year or more and probably do 2–3 higher-intensity exercise sessions (such as a gym class, running or cycling) a week.

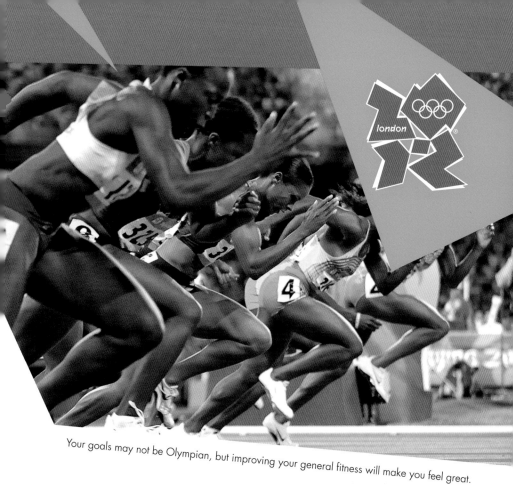

Your goals may not be Olympian, but improving your general fitness will make you feel great.

Make your lifestyle work for you. Sticking with the *Get fit for the Games* programmes will undoubtedly improve your strength, flexibility and endurance levels. But the amount of activity you fit into the rest of your life also matters. Studies have shown that any activity that raises your heart rate and gets you moving – from gardening and housework to an active commute – will contribute considerably towards your fitness. Indeed, researchers in the Netherlands found that people who led generally active lifestyles burned more calories on a daily basis than gym members who slotted in a short, sharp workout during their lunch hour or after work. The reason? After a hard bout of exercise, the gym-goers typically limited their physical activity for the rest of the day. The message is to integrate activity into your life whenever you can – at work, at home and when you socialise – for a fitter, more fabulous you.

Warming up and cooling down

Warming up and cooling down are the bookends of any workout, the fitness components that ensure the body is physically and mentally ready to start and finish an exercise session. Athletes would not consider launching into a training session without first preparing their body with a thorough warm-up lasting 10 minutes or longer.

A good warm-up should achieve two things: literally warm up the body to increase blood flow and loosen the muscles to prepare them for activity. Warm muscles pull oxygen from the bloodstream more easily and trigger the chemical reactions needed to produce energy more efficiently. Such preparation needn't take long, indeed, a warm-up that is too lengthy or vigorous will simply leave you feeling tired before you even get going.

Warming up

Around 10 minutes of jogging or brisk walking is the best way to get ready for a workout. At home, try walking up and down stairs for five minutes, marching on the spot or skipping (in a room where there are no low hanging light fittings). Some stretching helps to mobilise joints and lengthen connective tissues, reducing the risk of injuries. But don't overdo it. Exercise scientists have shown that too much 'static stretching' – the kind in which you hold a position for several seconds – can be detrimental if performed before a workout. Focus instead on 'dynamic' movements (such as arm swings and knee raises) that better prepare your body for what follows.

Cooling down

When it comes to cooling down, the important thing is never to stop

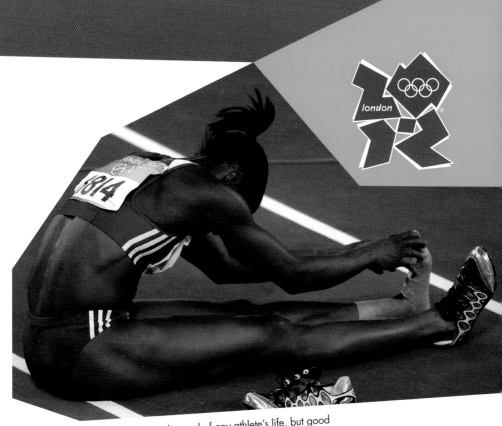

Injuries are part and parcel of any athlete's life, but good warm ups and cool downs will reduce their likelihood.

intense exercise abruptly. During exercise, the heart pumps faster and blood vessels expand to promote blood flow to the legs and feet. If you stop too suddenly blood can start to pool in the lower limbs, causing dizziness. Ideally, you should spend the last five minutes of a workout doing the same activity at a slower pace. If you haven't been exercising at a high intensity, then just walking around is fine.

A popular misconception is that cool-down stretches will stop muscles from becoming sore by flushing out lactic acid, the waste product of exercise. But since soreness is caused by minor damage to muscle fibres during exercise, stretching will have no effect on this particular problem. However, static stretches are best performed when muscles are warm, making the cool-down a good time to improve overall flexibility.

Spinal rotation

What it does:
Loosens the spine and the muscles around the torso.

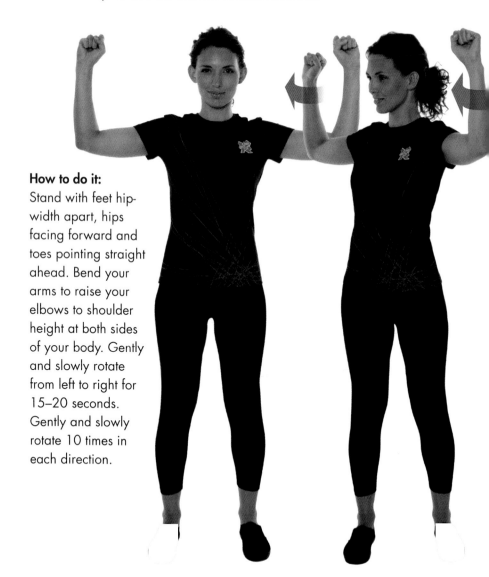

How to do it:
Stand with feet hip-width apart, hips facing forward and toes pointing straight ahead. Bend your arms to raise your elbows to shoulder height at both sides of your body. Gently and slowly rotate from left to right for 15–20 seconds. Gently and slowly rotate 10 times in each direction.

Chest stretch

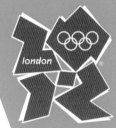

What it does:
Stretches the chest and shoulder muscles.

How to do it:
Stand with feet hip-width apart and hips facing forward. Clasp your hands together behind your back, keeping your arms straight. Gently raise your clasped hands upwards until you feel a stretch. Hold for 20 seconds, then lower your arms back down.

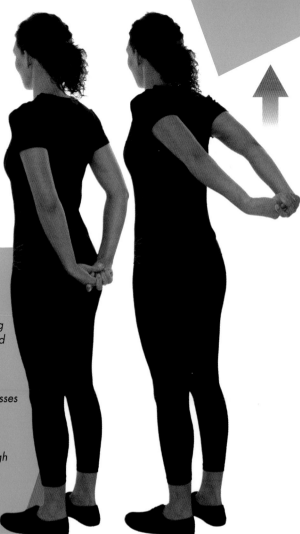

Did you know?
Regularly stretching the shoulder and chest muscles is particularly important if you spend a lot of time sitting down. Breathing is hampered as the body struggles to fill the lungs with oxygen when crunched in a seated position. Sitting also compresses the abdominal contents and digestion is slowed down as a result. All of this means energy levels can flag through lack of oxygen and sports performance is adversely affected. Stretch to undo the damage of sitting.

Side arm stretch

What it does:
Loosens the muscles in the waist and torso.

How to do it:
Stand with feet wider than shoulder-width apart, keeping your back straight and your chest lifted. Bend your knees slightly. Place your right hand on your right hip and stretch your left hand over your head. Lift from the waist and lean to the right without bending forward. Hold for 8–10 seconds and return to the start before repeating on the other side. Perform 6 stretches to each side.

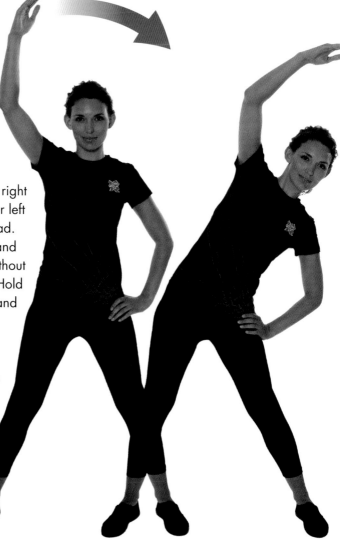

Arm swing

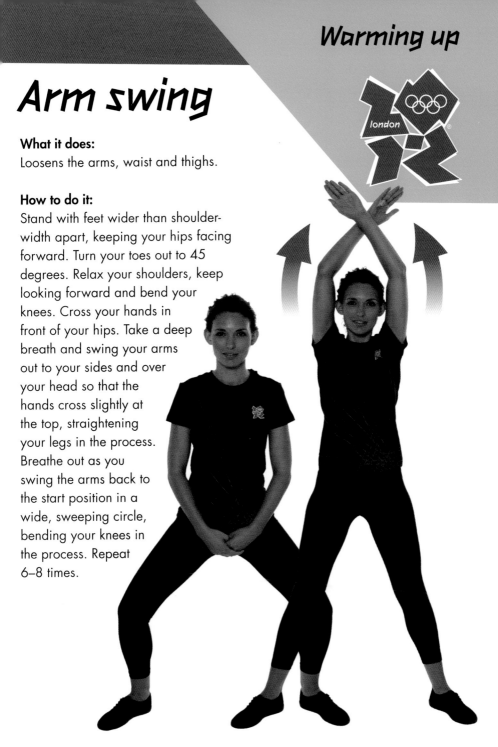

What it does:
Loosens the arms, waist and thighs.

How to do it:
Stand with feet wider than shoulder-width apart, keeping your hips facing forward. Turn your toes out to 45 degrees. Relax your shoulders, keep looking forward and bend your knees. Cross your hands in front of your hips. Take a deep breath and swing your arms out to your sides and over your head so that the hands cross slightly at the top, straightening your legs in the process. Breathe out as you swing the arms back to the start position in a wide, sweeping circle, bending your knees in the process. Repeat 6–8 times.

Knee raises

What it does:
Loosens the hamstrings at the back of the leg, the quadriceps at the front and the hip flexors.

How to do it:
Stand upright with feet hip-width apart and hands by your sides. Bend your right knee up towards your chest in a single, sweeping movement. Keep the foot flexed, not pointed. Then, keeping your arms in a running motion, lift your right foot up towards your bottom, again keeping the foot flexed rather than pointed. Repeat on the other side. Repeat 6–8 times on each leg.

Did you know?
Tightness in the hamstrings and hip flexor muscles can pull the back out of alignment and weaken its muscles. Perform this exercise regularly to stay loose.

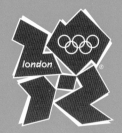

Standing quad stretch

What it does:
Stretches the quadriceps muscles in the front of the thigh.

How to do it:
Stand with feet hip-width apart, hips facing forward. Place your weight on the right foot, bend your left foot backwards and clasp it with your left hand behind you. Gently and slowly pull the left foot towards the buttocks, pointing the knee down as you do so. Repeat 3–5 times on each leg.

Did you know?
For a deeper stretch, try pushing the hips further forward.

Professional recovery techniques

How quickly athletes' bodies recover from a training session or competition determines how soon they can return to full training. Cooling down thoroughly and stretching regularly are essential, but athletes go to even greater lengths to speed up their return to exercise. Here are some of the methods they use.

Massage

Olympic swimmer Rebecca Adlington is one of many athletes who swear by regular deep-tissue massage to aid recovery. Registered sports massage therapists claim it increases blood flow to aching muscles and flushes out metabolic waste products, such as lactic acid, after a hard workout. Massage is also thought to reduce the swelling of tissues and aid minor soft-tissue injuries. Waiting until the day after a strenuous workout before having a massage is advised.

Ice baths

Taking a dip in a bathtub filled with ice-cold water is among the hottest therapies in top-level sport. When ice cools the body part it is applied to, the body senses the temperature drop and sends more blood supply to the area, boosting circulation and speeding up healing. Tiny tears occur to muscle fibres after a hard workout and ice can help to heal them. However, you don't need to raid the freezer to get the benefits. Physiotherapists say a cool shower or bath after a workout can also be helpful.

Recovery foods

What you eat after a workout can have a direct influence on your rate of recovery. Sports nutritionists who work with elite athletes focus as much on planning the post-training diet as they do on preparing a pre-competition menu. In prolonged endurance events like cycling, triathlons and marathons, the muscle stores of glycogen, the body's source of fuel for activity, become depleted after the race. They need to be replaced by consuming 0.5 gram of carbohydrate for every 2.2kg of your bodyweight – the equivalent of a bowl of breakfast cereal and a banana or a couple of sandwiches – 2–3 hours after the finish.

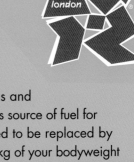

Compression garments

Members of Britain's Olympic and Paralympic teams will each be issued with items of team kit made from compression fabrics constructed from strong, supportive webbing material. They are designed not only to provide support to the muscles used in exercise but also to prevent excessive muscle vibration, which is thought to contribute to early-onset fatigue. One study in the *Journal of Science and Medicine in Sport* showed that sprinters who wore compression socks during training had less post-workout muscle soreness than those who wore ordinary socks.

Hydrotherapy

Hydrotherapy – the use of warm water and water jets to aid muscle recovery – is a practice favoured by many sports people. One study of Finnish athletes found that just 20 minutes of warm underwater massage using the jets in a spa helped athletes to maintain leg explosiveness and power the next day. Some swimming pools now have hydrotherapy suites, but physiotherapists claim that alternating warm and cool water jets in a shower can also be helpful.

Adductor stretch

What it does:
Stretches the adductor muscles in the inner thigh.

How to do it:
Sit on the floor with your back straight and put the soles of your feet together on the floor. Hold your ankles and gently press down on the inside of your knees with your elbows. Lean slightly forward from the hips and hold for 8–10 seconds.

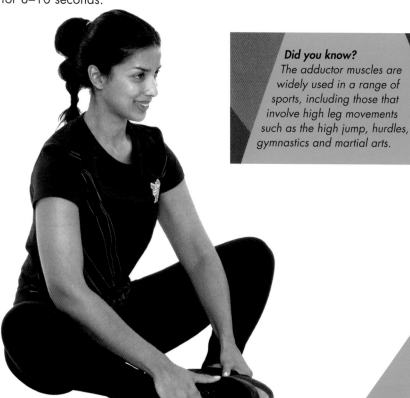

Did you know?
The adductor muscles are widely used in a range of sports, including those that involve high leg movements such as the high jump, hurdles, gymnastics and martial arts.

Calf stretch

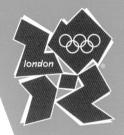

What it does:
Stretches the calf muscles in the back of the legs.

How to do it:
Stand with your hands on your hips, feet hip-width apart, and take a large step back with your right foot. Bend your left knee slightly but straighten your right leg, making sure both feet are facing forward. To feel the stretch, really push down on the back heel. Repeat 3–5 times on each leg.

Did you know?
Calf muscles become tired and stiff after prolonged bouts of running, not only in athletics events but in football, hockey and tennis matches. Failure to stretch them can lead to injury in the long term.

Waist twists

What it does:
Stretches the core
and waist muscles.

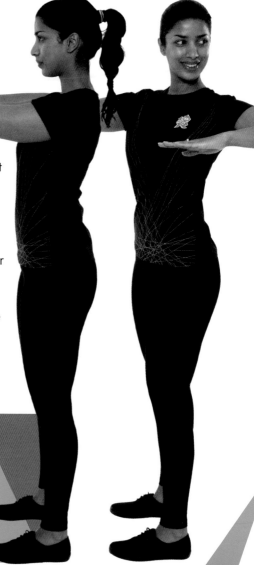

How to do it:
Stand with your back straight
and feet hip-width apart,
knees slightly bent. Reach
both arms out in front of you
at shoulder height. Bend
your left elbow and twist your
head and upper body as far
to the left as you can. Make
sure your hips remain square
to the front. Return to the
start position and repeat
on the other side.

Did you know?
*The waist is often ignored,
but its muscles are engaged
in many sports, especially
those that involve bending
and twisting at the waist
such as hockey, canoeing,
synchronised swimming,
rowing and wrestling.*

Triceps stretch

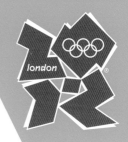

What it does:
Stretches the triceps muscles in the back of the arms.

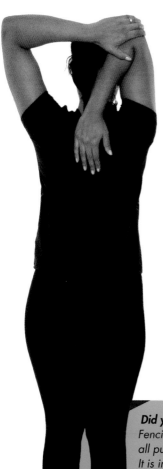

How to do it:
Stand with feet hip-width apart and hips square to the front. Bend your knees slightly and raise your right arm to bend at the elbow over your right shoulder. Pull your right elbow downwards with your left hand. Aim to touch between your shoulder blades with your right hand. Don't move your head during the stretch – keep your back straight. Repeat on the other side.

Did you know?
Fencing, handball, volleyball and archery all put a lot of strain on the tricep muscles. It is important to stretch the arms as often as you can throughout the day.

Stretching and flexibility

Our bodies are designed to be flexible, to respond to the demands placed on them by moving freely and efficiently. With good flexibility comes good posture and, in turn, unencumbered breathing and energy levels that soar. In this chapter, are a range of stretching exercises designed to keep your entire body supple and mobile, increasing its resistance to injury and enabling you to carry out everyday tasks with greater ease.

Like other aspects of fitness, flexibility training requires consistency of effort to produce results. The stretching and flexibility programme is designed to be done in its entirety 2–3 times a week, always preceded by a warm up. However, it is better to do some stretching than none and, if you lack time, select some of the stretches to perform after your Bronze, Silver or Gold workout, when your body temperature is raised and your muscles are warm. Another good idea is to pick a time of the day when you can multi-task by stretching when you are doing something else, such as watching the news or having a lunch break, or just before you go to bed.

Each of the exercises in this section is a 'static stretch', the kind in which you hold a position for several seconds in order to improve what physiologists call your passive range of motion, or the ability to stretch a muscle around a joint. Static stretching is very important for maintaining good posture and helping muscles to recover from exercise. However, as gentle as stretching seems, it is not without risk, so make sure you read the stretching guidelines that follow before you start.

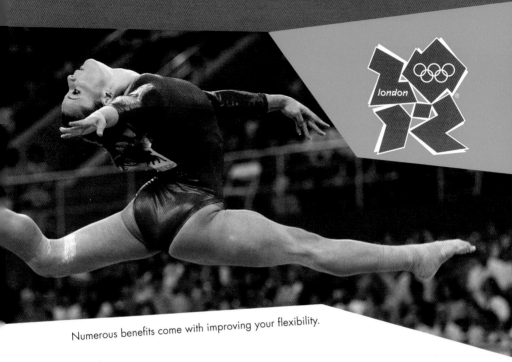

Numerous benefits come with improving your flexibility.

How to stretch:

- Never stretch cold muscles. Think of your muscles as being like rubber bands: if you put them in the freezer and leave them there for a while, then take one out and stretch it, it will snap; but if you warm it up in your hands you can stretch it and it will be a lot harder to snap.
- Don't stretch to the point of pain. When you reach the limit of your range of flexibility, you should feel slight discomfort, but a stretch should not be painful.
- Perform stretches in a slow and controlled manner – don't use jerky or forceful movements.

- Focus on technique and good posture – practise in front of a mirror if necessary.
- When a muscle is stretched to its limits, it triggers a 'stretch reflex' in which a nerve signals the muscle to contract – this is the body's automatic protective mechanism. Holding a stretch at this point for 8–10 seconds helps to override the stretch reflex so that you should eventually be able to stretch a little further with no pain. Gradually increase until you can hold each stretch for a further 15 seconds.

Full body stretch

What it does:
Stretches and loosens the major muscles all over the body, particularly those in the spine.

How to do it:
1. Lie on your front on the floor. Reach your arms out in front of you and gently stretch your entire body, imagining you are lengthening yourself from fingers to toes. Keep your hips pressed into the floor. Hold the stretch for 20 seconds. Gently bring your arms back to the start position.

Loosen up

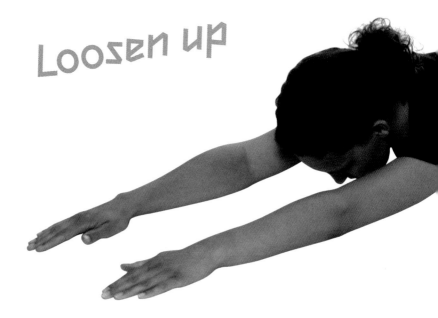

Stretching and flexibility

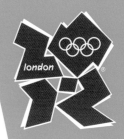

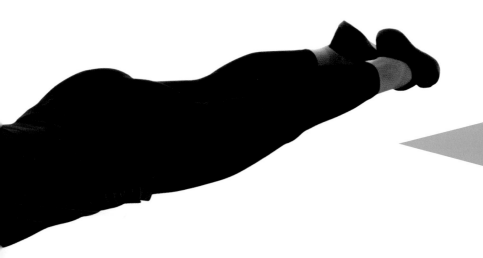

Top tip
Try the **Full body stretch** on your back, allowing your back to come slightly off the floor, but not arching it too much.

Lying crossed gluteal stretch

What it does:
Stretches the gluteal (or buttock) muscles as well as the upper leg.

How to do it:
1. Lie on your back with both knees bent and feet flat on the floor. Press your lower back into the floor and keep your shoulders relaxed. Cross your left foot over your right knee.

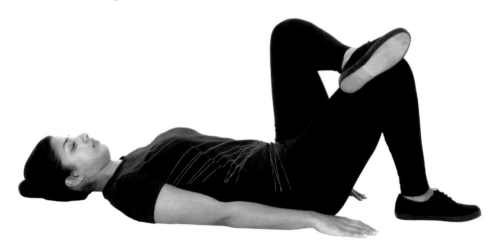

Take it slow

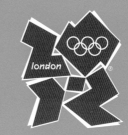

2. Slowly raise your right foot off the floor, bringing your
knees towards your chest in that position. When you
feel mild tension in the gluteal muscles, hold the stretch
for 8–10 seconds. Repeat on the other side.

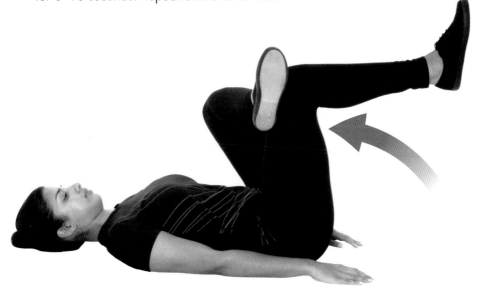

Upper back stretch

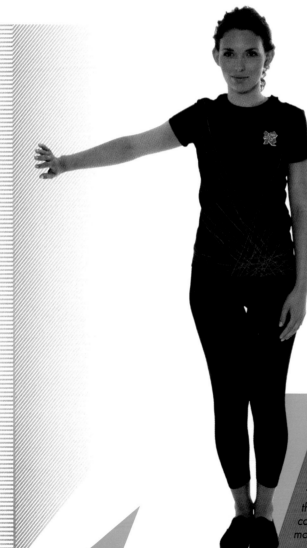

What it does:
Stretches the upper back and shoulders.

How to do it:

1. Stand about 60cm away from a wall with your right side facing it. Keep your back straight and hips facing forward. Place your feet together and bend your knees slightly. Keep your head upright. Place your right hand on the wall, with fingers facing forward, positioned at shoulder height.

Did you know?
Many sports include elements of bending, throwing and over-reaching with the upper body that can put strain on the shoulders and upper back. This stretch is great for releasing the tension that such movements cause and increasing range of movement in the upper back area.

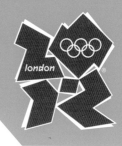

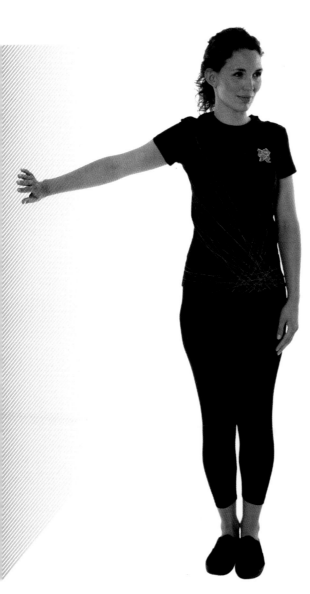

2. Keeping your hand on the wall, push forward with your right shoulder. Keep your elbow slightly bent – don't let it lock. Hold for 8–10 seconds. Repeat on the other side.

Forearm and wrist stretch

What it does:
Stretches the muscles in the wrist and forearm that can become stiff with computer use.

How to do it:
1. Reach both arms out in front of you. Turn the right hand and fingers upwards and use the left hand to pull the fingers gently towards the body and hold for 8–10 seconds. Repeat on your other hand.

Did you know?
The wrists are an often-neglected body part when it comes to training programmes. However, they play a crucial role in many sports, particularly martial arts, gymnastics, diving and hockey, and it is important to devote time to strengthening and stretching this area.

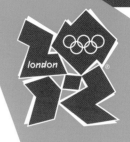

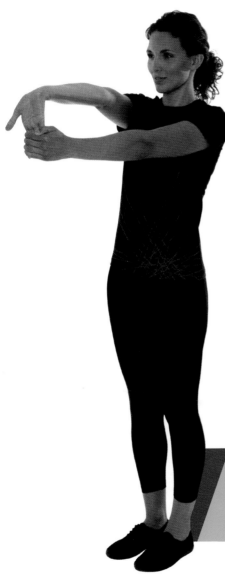

Be Flexible

2. Next, extend the arms, pointing the fingers downwards and gently pull the fingers to feel the stretch and hold for 8–10 seconds.

Top tip
The forearm and wrist stretch can be performed standing or sitting.

Hamstring stretch

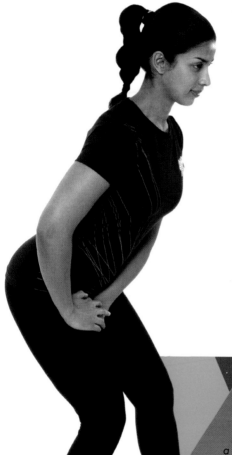

What it does:
Stretches the hamstring muscles in the back of the thigh.

How to do it:
1. Stand with feet hip-width apart, feet facing forward. Take a small step forward with your left leg and bend your right knee, keeping your feet flat on the floor. Place your hands on your right thigh.

Did you know?
Cyclists and triathletes love this stretch. Because of their riding position in the saddle and the pedalling action, their hamstrings have a tendency to tighten, which, over time, can cause problems such as back pain. This exercise helps to loosen and lengthen the hamstring muscles.

Hold it

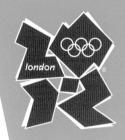

2. Lean forward from the hips, keeping your back straight and your head in line with your spine. Lower your upper body towards your left thigh. Hold the stretch for 20–30 seconds. Repeat on the other side.

Too easy?
To make the stretch more intense, flex the foot of your extended leg towards your body.

Five more ways exercise benefits body and mind

Exercise is like eating fruit and vegetables – everybody knows it's good for them, but they often fall short when it comes to getting enough. However, if inspiration is what you need, then there is plenty to support the notion that exercise does more than whittle away your waistline. Here are five reasons to stick with your workout programme.

It burns fat (even after you finish)

Fit people have more fat-burning molecules in their blood after exercise than people who work out infrequently. Analysis of blood taken before, just following and after healthy participants ran on a treadmill for 10 minutes showed that those with a relatively good level of fitness had a 98 per cent increase in their body's ability to break down stored fat, sugar and amino acids, compared with a 48 per cent rise in the less fit.

It fights disease

There is little doubt that active women are less prone to a host of diseases, including breast and other forms of cancer, heart disease, diabetes and the bone-thinning disease, osteoporosis. Simply integrating 30 minutes of activities like walking, doing the housework and climbing the stairs every day will see your risk of disease fall, but the more exercise you do, the greater the benefits become.

It could extend your life

Sorry couch potatoes, but people who work out really do live longer. In fact, those who get a good workout almost daily can add nearly four years to their life. American researchers found people who engaged in moderate activity – the equivalent of walking for 30 minutes a day for five days a week – lived about 1.3 to 1.5 years longer than those who were less active. Those who took on more intense exercise – the equivalent of running or cycling half an hour a day five days every week – extended their lives by about 3.5 to 3.7 years. A report in the *Journal of the American Heart Association* found that top athletes produce enzymes during exercise that have an anti-ageing effect at cellular level.

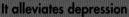

It alleviates depression

There is increasing evidence of a link between regular activity and improved mental health. Half an hour of exercise a day, six days a week, had effects equivalent to a course of prescribed medication for mildly depressed patients, according to one major study. Exercise is known to raise the brain's levels of dopamine, serotonin and norepinephrine, all neurotransmitters that affect mood. These are the same chemicals that are controlled by antidepressant medications.

It boosts your brainpower

Regular exercisers have been shown in various trials to outperform couch potatoes in tests of memory recall and mental agility. It is thought that activity boosts brainpower by building new brain cells in a brain region called the dentate gyrus, which is linked with memory and memory loss, and also that it improves circulation and oxygen supply to the grey matter.

Neck and shoulder stretch

What it does:
Stretches the main muscles in the neck and shoulders.

How to do it:
1. Stand with feet hip-width apart, back straight and abdominal muscles tucked in. Bend your knees slightly and place your hands behind your back. Keep your shoulders relaxed and your hips facing forward.

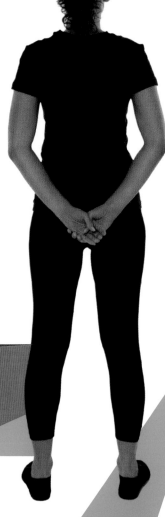

Did you know?
When stretching your neck and shoulders, you should never throw your head back as it puts pressure on the back of your neck and strain on the vertebrae at the top of the spine.

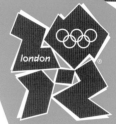

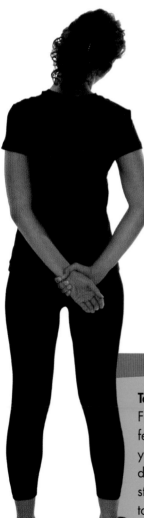

2. Lightly clasp your left wrist in your right hand and then lower your right ear towards your shoulder in a gentle movement. As you do this, gently pull your left wrist downwards so that you can feel a stretch in the neck area. Hold for 8–10 seconds. Let go of your wrist and then slowly return your neck to the start position. Repeat on the other side.

Too hard?

For an easier version of the neck stretch, stand with feet hip-width apart and knees slightly bent. Allow your hands to hang loosely at your sides and gently drop your left ear towards your left shoulder. Hold the stretch but don't move your shoulder or back. Return to the start position and repeat on the other side.

Cat stretch

What it does:
A yoga-inspired stretch for the shoulders and oblique muscles that run down the side of your trunk.

How to do it:
1. Kneel on the floor with knees hip-width apart. Slide your arms out in front of you, placing palms on the floor. Keep your buttocks slightly raised and your back flat.

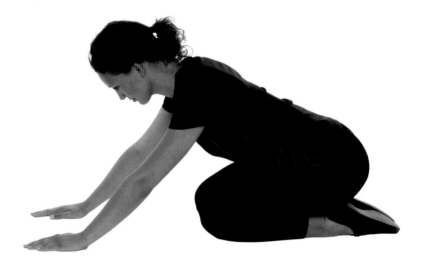

Too hard?
Another way to stretch the same muscles is to stand with feet hip-width apart and, keeping your head in line with the spine, reach as high as you can into the air with your arms.

Stretching and flexibility

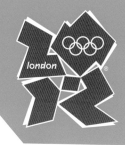

2. Imagine pressing your armpits into the floor, reaching as far forward with your hands as you can. Keep your head down and in line with your spine. At the point you feel mild tension in your spine, hold the stretch for 8–10 seconds. Slowly recoil to the start position.

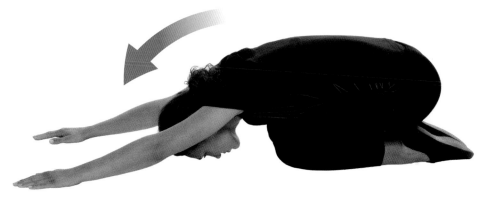

Back curl

What it does:
Stretches the entire spine.

How to do it:
1. Lie on the floor on your side. Draw your knees towards your chest as if you are scrunching your body into a tight ball. Keep your head on the floor, but in line with your spine. The aim is to curl up tightly by pulling your knees in as far as you can for maximum effect. Hold the stretch for 15–20 seconds, breathing normally throughout.

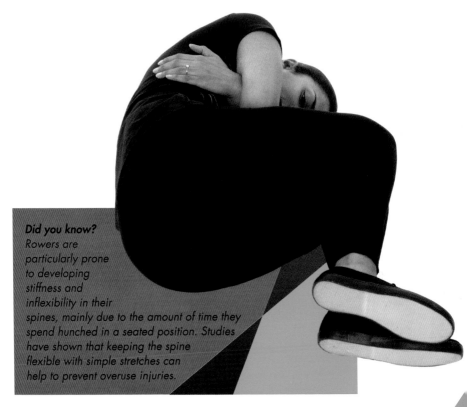

Did you know?
Rowers are particularly prone to developing stiffness and inflexibility in their spines, mainly due to the amount of time they spend hunched in a seated position. Studies have shown that keeping the spine flexible with simple stretches can help to prevent overuse injuries.

Cobra stretch

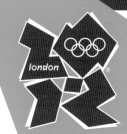

What it does:
Stretches the rectus abdominus muscles
in the front of the trunk.

How to do it:
1. Lie face down on the floor with legs together
   and hips pressed into the floor. Bend your
   arms at the elbow and place your forearms
   and palms flat on the floor, about shoulder-
   width apart and with elbows directly beneath
   the shoulders.
2. Exhale and slowly raise your upper body,
   pushing from the hands. Push as high as
   you can until the arms are almost straight
   (the movement should be slow and graceful,
   not forced). Relax your lower back and
   bear the weight on your arms without
   locking the elbows – keep your buttock
   muscles relaxed. Hold for 5–10 seconds
   before slowly lowering back down.
   Repeat 3–5 times.

Knee hug

What it does:
Stretches the gluteal muscles in the buttocks
and the thighs.

How to do it:

1. Lie on your back, knees bent and lifted towards your
chest. Place your hands behind your knees to pull
your legs in. Keep your lower back pressed into the
ground and your shoulders relaxed. Do not twist or
roll your head.

Did you know?
If this stretch is too intense, you can get an
effective stretch by sticking to the first phase of
the move and simply drawing the knees into the
chest by pulling behind the knees.

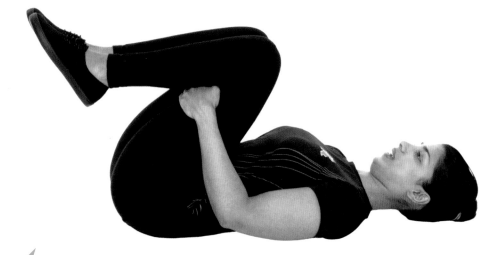

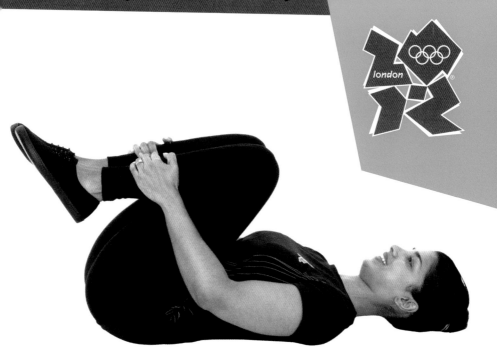

2. Place your hands on top of your shins towards your feet. Slowly draw your knees towards your chest. At the point where you feel tension in your buttocks, hold the stretch for 15–20 seconds.

Feel it working

Seated
shoulder stretch

What it does:
Stretches the anterior deltoid muscles in the shoulders
and the pectoral muscles in the chest.

How to do it:
1. Sit on the floor with legs stretched out in
   front of you, feet flexed. Support yourself
   with hands placed behind you, palms flat
   on the floor and fingers pointing away from
   your body. Keep your elbows slightly bent
   and your head straight, eyes facing forward.

Did you know?
An easier version of this exercise can be
performed by sitting with knees bent and feet flat
on the floor. As you become more flexible, gradually
lower your knees until they are stretched out in front of you.

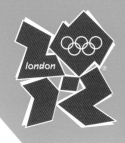

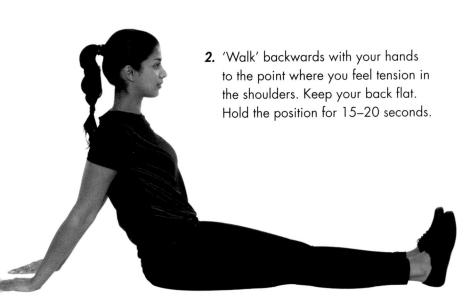

2. 'Walk' backwards with your hands to the point where you feel tension in the shoulders. Keep your back flat. Hold the position for 15–20 seconds.

stretch yourself

Forearm stretch

What it does:
Stretches the muscles in the forearms.

How to do it:

1. Kneel on all fours with your back straight and your head in line with the spine. Place the palms of your hands flat on the floor with fingers facing the body. Make sure your arms are directly in line with your shoulders. Lean back slowly and gently from the hips – this should be a very slight movement. When you feel tension in the forearms, hold the stretch for 10–15 seconds.

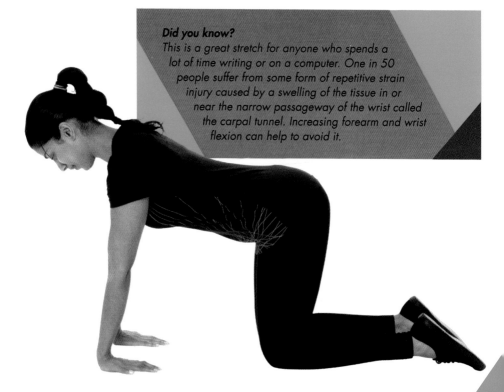

Did you know?
This is a great stretch for anyone who spends a lot of time writing or on a computer. One in 50 people suffer from some form of repetitive strain injury caused by a swelling of the tissue in or near the narrow passageway of the wrist called the carpal tunnel. Increasing forearm and wrist flexion can help to avoid it.

Lower back stretch

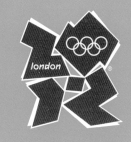

What it does:
Stretches and releases the lower back.

How to do it:

1. Lie face down and keep your hands by your
shoulders as if you are doing a press-up. Point your
toes downwards, as this helps to lengthen your spine.
Very slowly push up your torso as far as is comfortable
or until your hips begin to rise of the floor. Keep
your elbows and upper arms no higher than a few
of inches off the floor. Take five seconds to reach the
top of the position; lower yourself down again at the
same speed. Repeat 3–5 times.

> **Did you know?**
> A healthy human spine has a natural
> S-shape, but too much sitting pushes the
> lower lumbar curve into more of a C-shape,
> so that the back and abdominal muscles
> designed to support the body are unused.
> Over time, the postural muscles become so
> weak that they are unable to support the
> spine effectively and back pain inevitably
> ensues. Regularly stretching the spine
> can help to counter these problems.

Hip flexor stretch

What it does:

Stretches all the main muscles in the thighs.

How to do it:

1. Kneel on all fours with hands facing forward. Bend and lift your right knee, keeping the knee slightly forward of the ankle. Your right foot should be flexed and toes touching the floor. Keep your hips square to the front.

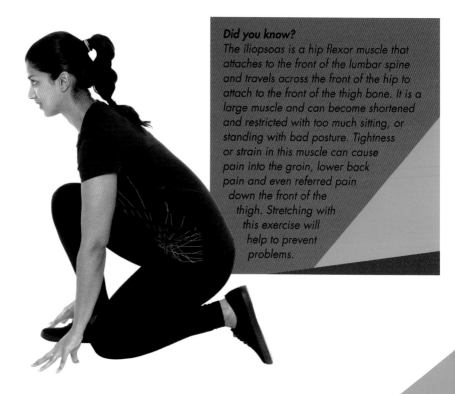

Did you know?
The iliopsoas is a hip flexor muscle that attaches to the front of the lumbar spine and travels across the front of the hip to attach to the front of the thigh bone. It is a large muscle and can become shortened and restricted with too much sitting, or standing with bad posture. Tightness or strain in this muscle can cause pain into the groin, lower back pain and even referred pain down the front of the thigh. Stretching with this exercise will help to prevent problems.

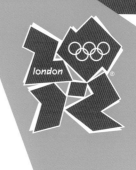

2. Slide your left leg back behind your body as far as you can, keeping your knee on the floor as you push back. Straighten the left leg so that the knee raises and the toes are flexed. Press forward and down from the hips. Keep your hands in position on the floor for support on the floor for support. Hold the stretch for 15–20 seconds at the point where you feel mild tension. Repeat on the other side.

Push yourself

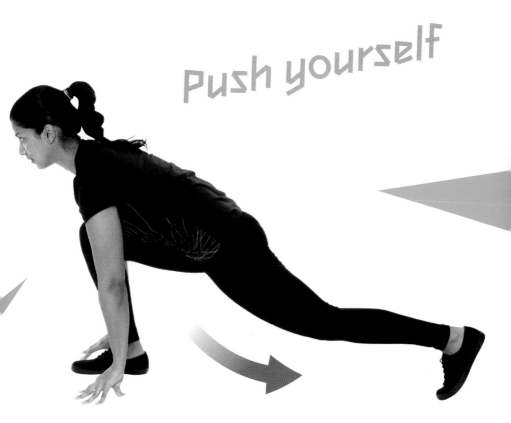

Stretching and flexibility – summary

Stretching can be performed before a one-off workout following a thorough warm-up or it can be slipped easily into your day. You can perform stretches at your desk, in front of the television or even when you are in the car. What matters, particularly as you are about to embark on an exercise programme, is that stretching becomes second nature, as much a part of your daily routine as brushing your teeth.

Any form of exercise that pushes the body beyond its comfort zone causes constant tightening and shortening of the muscles. This effect is beneficial in terms of improving your overall fitness. Unless you stretch regularly, there is a risk that the muscles you have been working remain contracted, becoming tight and less efficient. Unless addressed, this can cause muscular imbalance as you over-rely on other muscles to compensate for the tightness in a particular area.

Our natural flexibility also declines as we get older – most people find they struggle to perform the stretches they did with ease when they were 20 by the time they are 35 or 40. Advancing age draws moisture and fluid from the collagen fibres within connective tissues and with soft tissues also becoming dehydrated, our joints are less well lubricated and our muscles stiffer. The more regularly and thoroughly you stretch, the better able your body will be to offset this downturn in flexibility.

Stretching does far more than improve your range of motion – it can help you to unwind mentally and to

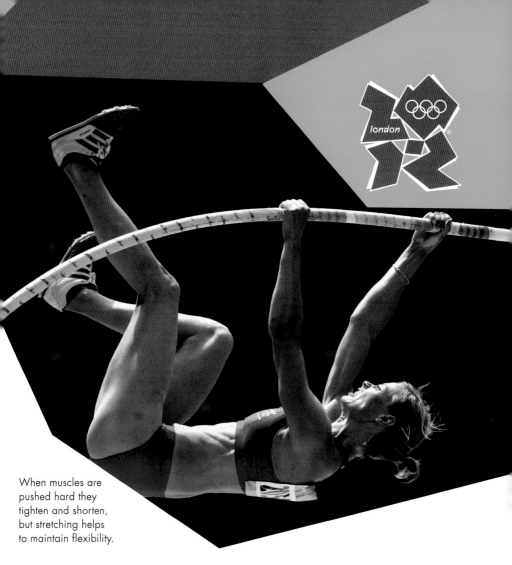

When muscles are pushed hard they tighten and shorten, but stretching helps to maintain flexibility.

relax after a tough day. Researchers at Louisiana State University showed that regular stretching workouts three times a week not only enhanced flexibility, but improved strength and endurance. Perhaps the biggest gains come in the form of improved posture. Our sedentary lifestyles mean we spend much of our time hunched in a seated position that shortens the hamstrings (at the back of the legs), the calf muscles, the chest muscles and the adductor muscles that pull the legs into the body. If your time is limited, concentrate on stretching these areas and watch your body lengthen, as it becomes less like a coiled spring.

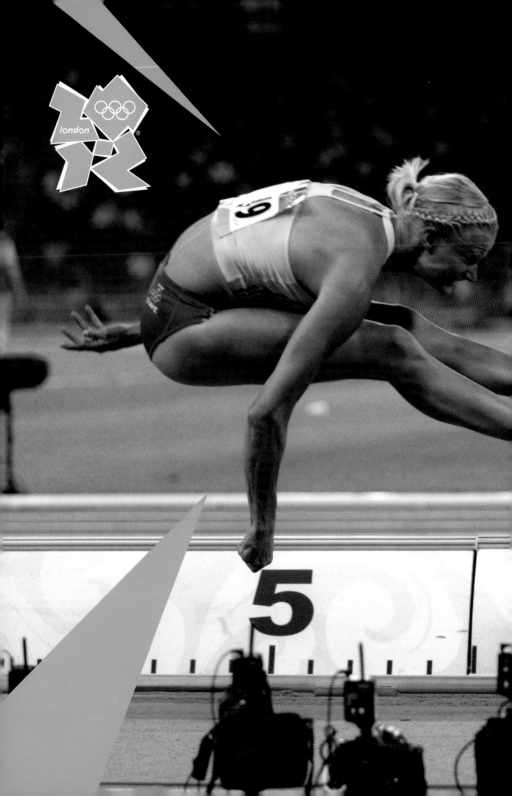

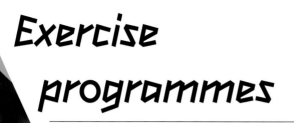

Exercise programmes

Now you are fully prepared to launch yourself into the starting blocks of the *Get fit for the Games* workout plans. Follow the appropriate programme and watch as your body is gradually transformed into a fitter, stronger version of its former self and revel in the mental boost that comes with pursuing your own take on Olympic or Paralympic glory.

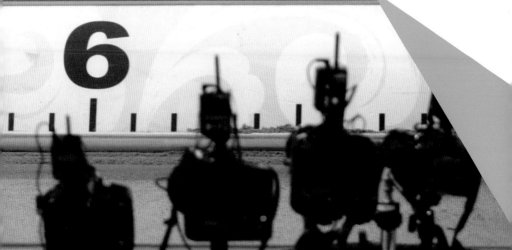

Olympians and Paralympians dedicate themselves to their sport, training for years to reach their optimum fitness. For most, competing in the Games marks the pinnacle of their career.

Bronze workout introduction

If you are new to exercise, or if you haven't worked out for a while, the prospect of launching head-first into a structured training regime may seem daunting. But even Olympians and Paralympians once had to start at the beginning and the hardest thing about getting fit is getting started.

The Bronze workout is designed to provide you with a gentle but effective step towards improved fitness and a healthier, better-functioning body and mind. Within the programme are exercises that will work every muscle group in your body. When muscle fibres are stimulated through activity, your metabolic rate is raised and you will burn more calories, eventually resulting in weight loss.

This 12-week plan is designed to be progressive, so that you increase the amount of work you do as you get fitter. Start by completing the workout twice a week, on non-consecutive days, gradually building up to three times a week by the end of the programme. If you find after week 2 that the workout is too strenuous, stay at that level for another week. Likewise, if some of the exercises begin to feel too easy, try the more advanced alternatives that are sometimes listed.

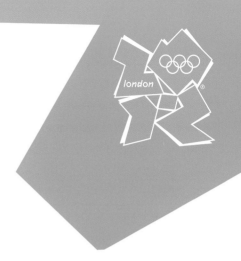

Get into it

Remember, too, that getting fitter is about changing your lifestyle, and the more time you devote to aerobic activity and stretching exercises each week, the better. Within weeks of starting the programme, you will find that your body image improves, along with your energy levels and sleep patterns. You will be in a better mood, feel less drained by the rigours of life and will start to notice changes for the better in your body shape and tone. What's to lose?

Bronze workout schedule

Always perform a thorough warm up and cool down before and after a workout. Take two minutes recovery between each set of exercises. On 2–3 other days a week, do 10–20 minutes of any aerobic activity – walking, cycling, swimming, running or indoor rowing. Try to set aside 15–30 minutes a week while watching television for stretching and flexibility.

Weeks	Repetitions	Weeks	Repetitions
1–2	1 set of 8 *(of each exercise)*	7–8	2 sets of 12
3–4	1 set of 12	9–10	3 sets of 10
5–6	2 sets of 8	11–12	3 sets of 12

Dumbbell curl

Work your bicep muscles as you lift in this exercise to maximise the strengthening and toning effect.

What it does:
Strengthens the biceps and other muscles in the front of the arm.

How to do it:

1. Stand with feet shoulder-width apart, knees slightly bent and hips facing forward. Hold a set of dumbbells or bottles of water in the underhand position (palms facing upwards). Keep your shoulders relaxed, back straight and head in line with the spine. Make sure your arms are tucked into your body. Bend your elbows slightly, but keep your wrists straight.

Did you know?
Lifting weights that are too heavy for your fitness level in this exercise will not lead to rapid improvements in strength but will simply place unnecessary strain on the upper body. Start with bottles of water or cans of beans and progress to using dumbbells only when you are strong enough, using 1–1.3kg weights at first.

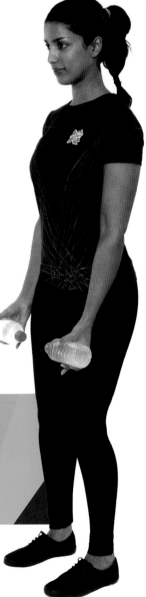

Bronze workout

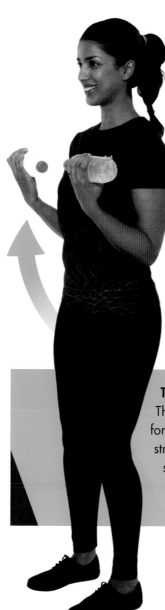

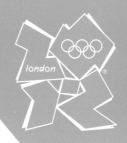

2. Exhale as you slowly raise the weights up towards your shoulders, making sure the upper arm remains close to the body at all times. Hold briefly at the top of the move before lowering the weights back down in a controlled manner.

Top tip

There's a natural tendency for the elbows to pull forward of the trunk as you get tired and this can strain the back. To avoid it, perform the exercise standing against a wall. Engage your core muscles to prevent the back from buckling under pressure.

Twists

Want to whittle away your waist? This is one of the best moves to get started.

What it does:
Strengthens the external oblique muscles in the abdominal area.

How to do it:
1. Lie on your back with knees bent and feet flat on the floor. Keep your head straight and gently place your hands at the sides of your head near your ears. Keep your elbows level – no higher than your ears – and make sure your lower back is pressed down. Cross your right foot over your left knee.

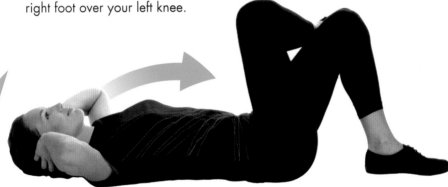

Too hard?
For an easier version of this exercise, take your left hand away from your head and extend your hand (rather than your elbow) towards your right knee. Repeat on the other side.

Bronze workout

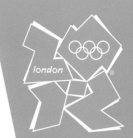

2. Exhale and slowly raise your left shoulder upwards and across your body towards your right knee. Keep your lower back on the floor – you should twist from the waist. Keep your right arm on the floor. At the top of the movement hold briefly before lowering back down in a controlled way, using your abdominal muscles for support. Complete a set on one side before changing to the other.

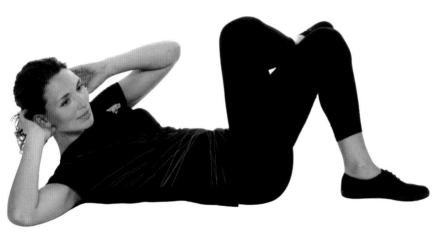

Did you know?
Britain´s double Olympic gold medalist Kelly Holmes said cashew nuts were her secret weapon in helping to boost her powers of recovery so she was fully primed for her Olympic finals. A 50g serving of cashews provides one-fifth of a woman´s daily iron requirements and is a rich source of dietary protein – needed to enhance the recovery process of muscles after intense activity.

Wall press-up

The beginner's version of the full press-up, which will help to tone the arms, chest and upper body.

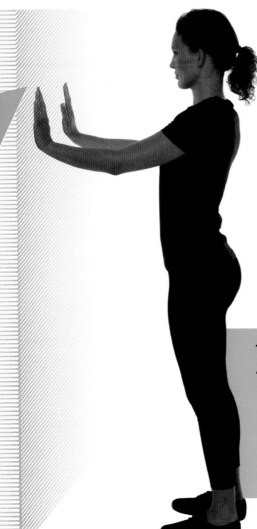

What it does:
Strengthens the shoulders, chest and triceps muscles in the back of the arms as well as the core muscles.

How to do it:
1. Stand facing a wall, about 60cm away from it. With feet hip-width apart and hips facing forward, place your hands flat on the wall in line with your shoulders, with fingers pointing upwards. Your hands should be positioned shoulder-width apart.

Too easy?
As you get stronger, progress to the **Box press-up** in the **Silver workout** on pages 132–133 and then the **Full press-up** in the **Gold workout** on pages 172–173.

Press on

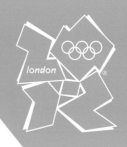

2. Breathe in and bend your arms at the elbows to lean your body towards the wall. Keep your back straight and your head in line with your spine. Try to touch the wall with your nose. Hold the position for a couple of seconds and breathe out as you press away from the wall with your arms.

Did you know?
The ability to do press-ups is considered an important indicator of the capacity to withstand ageing. Researchers have noted that press-ups can provide the strength and muscle memory needed to reach out and break a fall. When elderly people fall forward, they instinctively reach out to try and prevent the fall, ending in a move that mimics the push-up. The hands hit the ground, the wrists and arms absorb much of the impact, and the elbows bend slightly to reduce the force. The better someone is at performing press-ups, the less likely they are to be injured as a result of a fall.

Beginner lower back raise

An entry-level version of a move designed to improve strength and posture.

What it does:
Strengthens the erector spinae muscles in the lower back.

How to do it:
1. Lie face down with legs stretched out and toes pointing downwards. Push your hips into the floor and rest your forehead on the floor. Place the palms of your hands on your buttocks and breathe in.

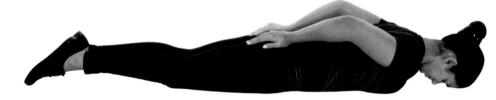

Did you know?
The key to this exercise is to make sure the movement is slow and controlled. Raising the upper body too high or too forcefully will cause strain and discomfort in the upper and lower back.

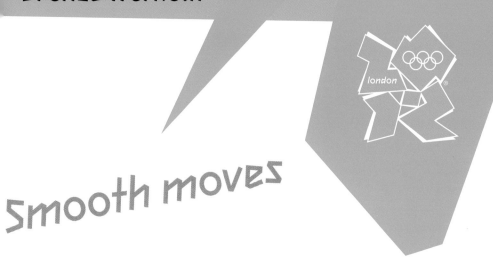

Smooth moves

Too easy?
If you find this exercise too easy, try **Intermediate lower back** raises in the **Silver workout** on pages 156–157.

2. As you exhale, slowly raise your upper body off the floor in a controlled and smooth movement. Hold briefly at the top of the move before lowering back down in a controlled manner.

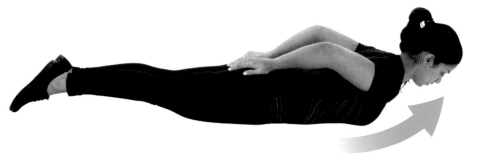

Beginner calf raise

Give your lower legs definition by performing this simple move as often as you can at home.

What it does:
Strengthens the calf muscles in the back of the lower leg.

How to do it:
1. Stand with back straight and hips facing forward, feet slightly wider than hip-width apart. Place your hands on the back of a dining chair for support. Keep your head in line with your spine and inhale.

Did you know?
This exercise is essential for any sport that involves running. Not only does it strengthen the calf muscles that provide some of the power for each running stride, but it also strengthens and stretches the Achilles tendon, which runs from the heel up through the leg and is prone to injury.

Bronze workout

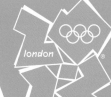

2. Exhale and press up onto the balls of your feet using your calf muscles. Hold the position when you are on tiptoes, squeezing the calf muscles for a couple of seconds. Breathe in and slowly lower back down to the start position.

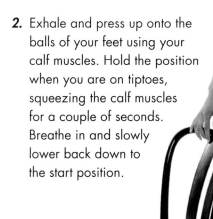

Beginner side leg lift

This is a great exercise for streamlining the thighs and developing strength in the upper leg.

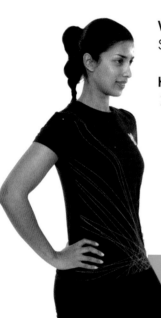

What it does:
Strengthens the adductor muscles in the outer thigh.

How to do it:
1. Stand at right angles to a step or raised platform. Place your left foot on the step and put your hands on your hips. Straighten your back and contract your abdominal muscles.

Did you know?
Strong abductor muscles cut the risk of injury from strenuous exercise and lessen muscle soreness. Although the hip abductor muscles work when performing exercises such as squats or lunges, they are often overlooked and it is a good idea to isolate and target them with exercises like this.

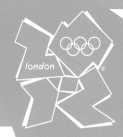

Too easy?
Try the advanced **Outer thigh lift** in
the **Gold workout** on pages 190–191.

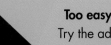

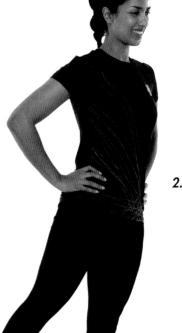

Keep going

2. Put your weight on your left foot
and raise your right leg out to the
side, lifting it as high as possible
while you maintain good balance.
Do not lean with your body. Lower
the leg back down to return to
the start position. Repeat before
switching sides.

Leg raise

This straightforward exercise tones the muscles in the upper leg.

What it does:
Strengthens the quadriceps muscles in the front of the thigh and the hamstring muscles in the back of the thigh.

How to do it:
1. Place your right foot on a low bench or the second step of a flight of stairs. Keep your back straight, place your hands on your hips and keep your abdominal muscles tucked in.

Did you know?
Sports that involve twisting, turning, and jumping, such as hockey and tennis, can play havoc with the knee joint, raising the risk of painful injuries such as tears of the anterior cruciate ligament. However, exercises that involve standing on one leg will help to strengthen the muscles at the front of the thigh that stabilise the knee joint.

2. Put the weight on your right foot and raise your left leg behind you, aiming to raise it as high off the ground as you can without arching the lower back. Keep your head in line with your spine. Hold the leg at its top height for 2–3 seconds before lowering to the start position. Perform an entire set on the left leg before switching to the right.

Balance

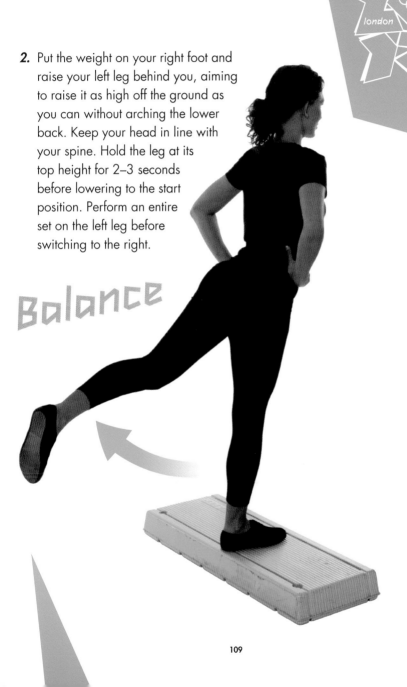

Five ways to improve your performance

Improving your fitness does not all boil down to hours spent exercising. Sometimes, tweaking various aspects of a workout regime can make a huge difference to your performance.

Perfect your timing

When you work out can make a difference to how you feel and perform. Research shows that late afternoon and early evening – when body temperature rises, warming the muscles and connective tissues – are the best times to exercise. In one study when people were asked to perform the same workout at different times of the day (5am, 11am, 5pm and 11pm), they felt they were working hardest first thing. It's no surprise, then, that most Olympic records are broken later in the day. But what if your lifestyle makes later workouts impossible? Find a time that works well for you and stick to it. American studies have shown that everyone, from novices to Olympians, benefits from working out at the same time each day.

Use a mirror

Poor technique is one of the main causes of workout injuries, but it will also reduce the efficiency of your exercise. A solution could be to work out in front of a mirror. A study in the *Journal of Medicine and Science in Sports and Exercise* found that newcomers to exercise benefited greatly from assessing their posture and technique in a mirror.

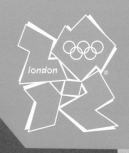

Take a rest

Intense, prolonged training or a sudden stepping up of workout frequency causes micro-tears to muscle fibres. As muscles mend – through rest – they become stronger. But if you tear those muscles again before they've fully recovered, you won't achieve your maximum potential. Researchers at Ball State University looked at the effects of rest on a group of novice athletes and found that both leg strength and performance plummeted in those who failed to take enough recovery time. Two days of active recovery (walking, gentle stretching) is recommended after a tough session.

Do more in less time

Research by the American College of Sports Medicine has shown that, often, people who spend lengthy periods working out simply clock up 'dead miles'. Exercising for 30 minutes at a fairly high intensity (that's at 80 per cent of your maximum aerobic capacity, a level at which you would be puffing and sweating) is as good as an hour at a workload of 60 per cent. Another study, published in the *Journal of Applied Physiology*, found people who reduced the overall volume of their workouts by 25 per cent could still improve their fitness as long as they added bursts of full-out effort.

Get tested

A battery of physiological and biomechanical tests are carried out on athletes. But assessments such as gait analysis (to test your running and walking posture for imbalances), VO_2 Max (your maximal oxygen uptake and an indicator of your aerobic fitness) and other assessments are available to the public at sports science laboratories around the country. Regular tests can also help you plot your progress.

Seated squat

Perform this move regularly and the result will be leaner, firmer and more toned thighs, buttocks and lower legs.

What it does:
Strengthens the quadriceps, hamstring and gluteal muscles in the front and back of the thighs and buttocks.

How to do it:
1. Stand with your back straight and feet wider than hip-width apart. Bend your knees slightly. Extend your arms out in front of you at or just below shoulder height and look directly ahead.

2. Inhale and bend from your knees and hips into a squat that is almost a seated position, with knees bent as close to right angles as possible. Keep your heels on the floor and the weight over your ankles for stability. Make sure your back is flat and your knees are in line with your feet; keep your shoulders forward of the mid-line of your thigh. Aim to get your thighs almost parallel with the floor if you can. Breathe out and, leading with your shoulders, slowly stand up.

Too easy?
Once you gain strength in your lower body, try adding light weights or holding bottles of water in each hand. Hold them close to your body at waist height as you squat.

Bronze workout

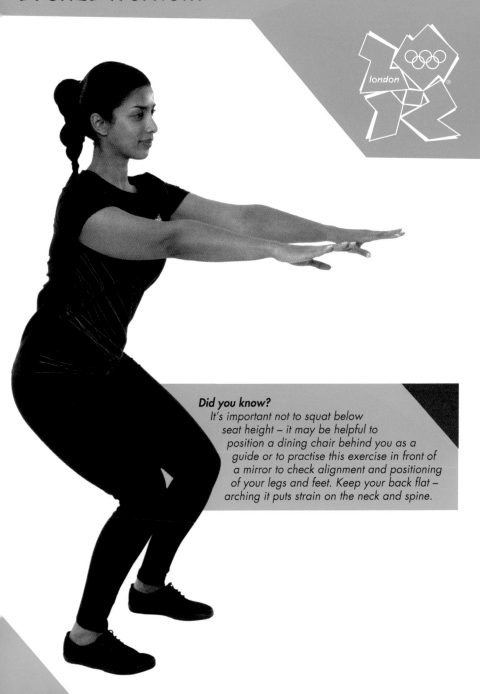

london

Did you know?
It's important not to squat below
seat height – it may be helpful to
position a dining chair behind you as a
guide or to practise this exercise in front of
a mirror to check alignment and positioning
of your legs and feet. Keep your back flat –
arching it puts strain on the neck and spine.

Can opener

So called because it simulates a can-opening action, this exercise both stretches and strengthens muscles in the hip area.

What it does:
Strengthens muscles in the outer thigh and loosens the hip flexors.

How to do it:
1. Lie on your side, supporting your head with your hand and bend your knees at 90 degrees towards your chest.

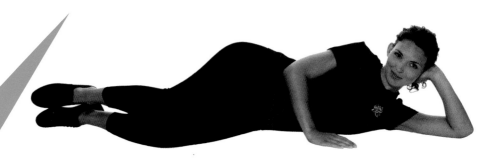

> **Did you know?**
> The hip flexors are the Iliopsoas major, Iliopsoas minor and Iliacus muscles. They lie deep on the lower abdomen, attached to the vertebral bones running over the inner surface of the pelvis, finally attaching to the inside of the upper thigh bones. These muscles work in conjunction with the groin muscles to pull the thigh towards the chest in order to lift the knee and are very important when running.

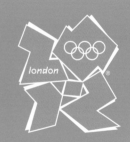

Enjoy it

What not to do: This exercise should not cause straining in the lower back. Stop at once if you feel pain.

2. Keep your feet together and open your knees, using your hips and feet as hinges. Pull your knees as far apart as you can while maintaining control and stability. Hold briefly at the top of the move before returning the legs slowly to the start position and repeating for a full set. Change sides.

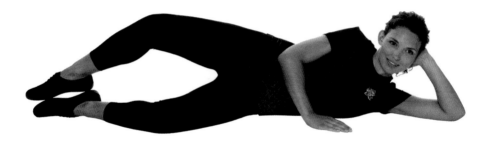

Beginner leg extension

Leaner looking thighs will be the result if you combine this move with plenty of aerobic activity.

What it does:
Works the quadriceps and hamstring muscles in the front and back of the thighs.

How to do it:
1. Lie on your back with arms at your sides and abdominal muscles tucked in. Press your lower back into the floor to prevent arching and look straight up at the ceiling. Slowly draw your knees towards your chest.

Too easy?
Try the **Advanced leg extension** in the **Gold workout** on pages 184–185.

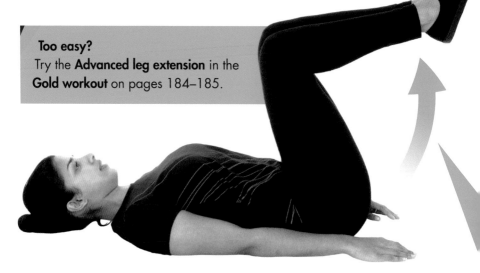

Bronze workout

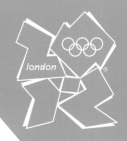
Did you know?
A lack of strength and flexibility in the hamstrings can leave the quadriceps to do more work, creating an imbalance in the legs. This can lead to straining or pulling of the hamstring muscle. Practise this move to strengthen the entire thigh.

Lift off

2. Raise your legs towards the ceiling by leading with your heels. Keep your feet flexed and your knees almost together. Don't let your knee joint lock. Hold the position at the top of the move. Slowly bend your legs and return to lower them down to the chest. Repeat.

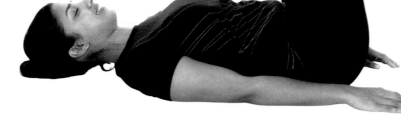

Shoulder press

This move can be performed standing or sitting, although you will reduce the work done by your abdominal muscles if you do it seated.

What it does:
Strengthens the deltoid and trapezius muscles in the upper back and shoulders, and the triceps muscles at the back of the arms.

How to do it:
1. Hold a set of light dumbbells or bottles of water at your sides. Stand with feet hip-width apart, knees bent, hips square to the front and back straight. Lift the weights to shoulder height with palms facing forward and elbows bent at 90 degrees. Keep your head in line with your spine. Contract your abdominal muscles and breathe in.

Top tip
If you perform this exercise sitting down, make sure your back is well supported.

Bronze workout

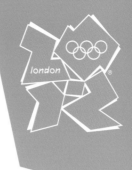

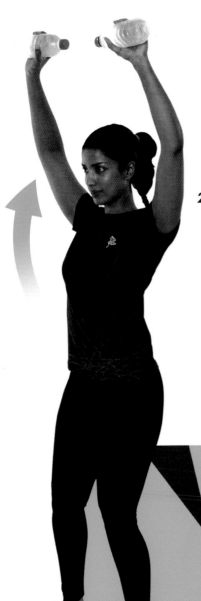

2. As you exhale, bend your elbows slightly and press the weights to almost arm's length above the head (don't lock your elbows), leading with your knuckles pointing towards the ceiling. Keep your back straight. At the top of the move, pause briefly before breathing in and lowering the weights back down to shoulder height. Repeat.

Did you know?
Improvements in muscle strength and tone occur more quickly in the upper body, according to research published in the European Journal of Applied Physiology. After 12 weeks of an all-over conditioning programme, a group of women improved upper body strength by up to 31 per cent, whereas muscle gains in the lower body were only 8 per cent.

Beginner hamstring curl

Take your time with this exercise – the movement should be controlled and executed without sudden jolts.

What it does:
Strengthens the hamstring muscles in the backs of the thighs and the gluteus maximus in the buttocks.

How to do it:
1. Lie face down on the floor, resting your head on your left forearm and stretching your right arm out in front of you. Press your hips into the floor and keep your knees level.

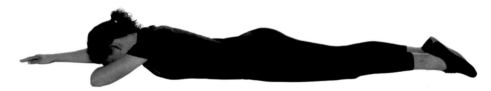

2. Flex your left foot and raise it about 5cm off the floor. Breathe in, then, as you breathe out, slowly curl your foot heel-first towards your buttocks. Keep your hips firmly on the floor. Hold the curl position briefly, breathe in and slowly lower your leg back to 5cm off the floor. Complete one set before changing legs.

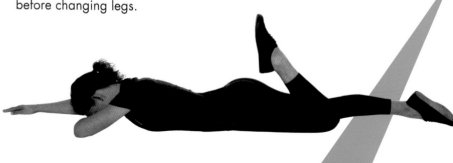

Beginner crunch

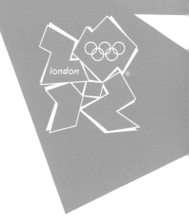

A wonderful exercise for toning your mid-section and stomach area.

What it does:
Works the rectus abdominus muscles in the abdomen.

How to do it:

1. Lie on your back with knees bent and hip-width apart and with your feet flat on the floor. Press your lower back into the floor and contract your abdominal muscles tightly. Place both hands on the front of your thighs. Breathe in.

2. As you exhale, slowly raise your shoulders off the floor in a small, controlled movement – the aim is not to lift them too far. Slide your palms up towards your knees, keeping your lower back down. Hold briefly at the top of the movement before lowering the shoulders down. Keep your abdominal muscles contracted throughout. Allow your shoulders to brush the floor before repeating the move.

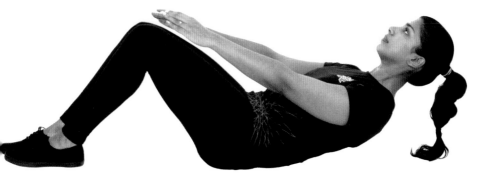

Shoulder shrug

A straightforward move that leads to toned shoulders and a strong upper back.

What it does:
Works the trapezius and rhomboid muscles in the upper back.

How to do it:
1. Stand with back straight and feet hip-width apart. Hold a set of light dumbbells or bottles of water in your hands with arms at your side and elbows relaxed. Bend your knees slightly. Keep your head in line with your spine and shoulders relaxed. Breathe in.

Did you know?
Swimmers are prone to an inflammatory injury dubbed 'swimmer's shoulder' that is caused by the repetitive overhead motion of the front crawl and other strokes. Exercises such as this one that strengthen the upper back and shoulders can help to prevent the kind of swimming posture that is susceptible to injury.

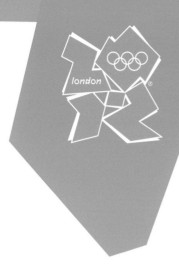

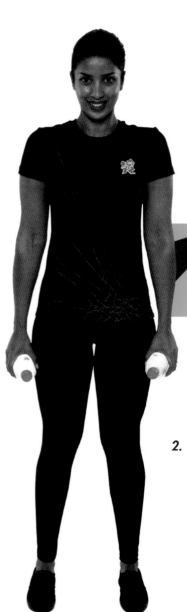

Too easy?
If you find this exercise too easy,
try the **Single arm row** in the
Silver workout on pages 160–161.

2. Exhale and slowly raise your
shoulders and roll them back.
Keep the weights close to your
sides at all times. Hold briefly
at the top of the move before
lowering your shoulders back to
the start position. Repeat.

Single arm crunch

A wonderful exercise for toning your mid-section and stomach area.

What it does:
Works the rectus abdominus muscle in the abdomen.

How to do it:
1. Lie on the floor with your knees bent and feet flat
on the floor. Keep your feet and knees hip-width
apart and press your lower back into the floor.
Place your hands lightly at the sides of your head.

Did you know?
*Elite athletes rarely suffer from a stitch when
they are training and it's mainly down to their
strong abdominal muscles. During exercise
our internal organs bounce up and down,
pulling on the diaphragm muscles. If this
tugging occurs when the diaphragm
moves upwards – or when we breathe
out – the strain is so great that it causes
a stitch. Exercises such as this one
can help to prevent the problem.*

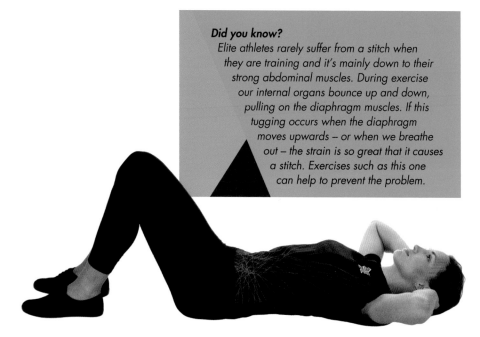

Bronze workout

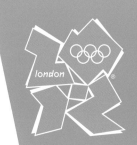

2. Contract your abdominal muscles and keep your head in line with your spine as you place your left hand behind your head (to cup it gently) and your right hand on the front of your right thigh. Take a deep breath and as you exhale slowly raise your shoulders off the floor to slide your right hand as close to your knee as you can. Throughout the move, keep your lower back pressed down and your left elbow back behind your head. Hold the position at the point where you can feel tension in your abdominal muscles. Breathe in and slowly lower yourself back down to the floor, using your abdominal muscles for control. Lightly touch the floor with your shoulders before repeating the move on the same side for 8–12 repetitions. Change sides.

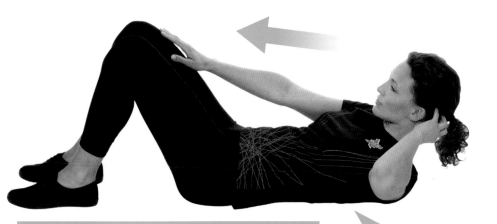

Too easy?
As you get stronger, aim to reach to an imaginary point just past your knee as you slide your hand forward.

Bronze workout
— summary

Throughout each of the workouts in this book, it's important to reassess your progress on a regular basis. When you have completed the 12-week Bronze workout, ask yourself whether you found the final two to four weeks tough going. If so, repeat them a second time to make sure you are ready to progress to the next level. Focus on improving exercises that you found particularly challenging and persevere until you can master them.

Suggested order of exercises

Ideally, the Bronze workout should be performed in its entirety, but all of the exercises can be mixed- and matched to suit your time constraints and personal needs. Try not to perform consecutive exercises on the same muscle groups. A good way to ensure you do this is by alternating upper- and lower- body moves and interspersing them with some exercises for the abdominal area. Here is a suggested order of routine, but it is not set in stone and can be changed according to your preference:

- Dumbbell curl (pages 96–97)
- Beginner hamstring curl (page 120)
- Twists (pages 98–99)
- Wall press-up (pages 100–101)
- Side leg lift (pages 106–107)
- Lower back raise (pages102–103)
- Beginner calf raise
  (pages 104–105)
- Leg raise (pages 108–109)
- Shoulder press (pages 118–119)
- Beginner leg extension (pages 116–11
- Can opener (pages 114–115)
- Beginner crunch (page 121)
- Seated squat (pages 112–113)
- Shoulder shrug (pages 122–123)
- Single arm crunch
  (pages 124–125)

Bronze workout

Are you working hard enough?

A useful gauge of effort is to calculate your Maximum Heart Rate (or MHR). To do this, subtract your age from 220 (a figure physiologists consider to be the average MHR of most people at birth). So, if you are 35, your MHR will be 185. As you work out, check your heart rate (see page 40 for how to do this), then refer to the table below to make sure you are working in the training zone of 65–75% of your MHR – that's a level that will see you breathing more heavily than usual, but still able to hold a conversation.

Age	65%	70%	75%	Age	65%	70%	75%
18–25	130	139	149	43–50	116	121	129
26–30	127	134	144	51–58	112	116	124
31–36	124	130	140	59–65	108	110	118
37–42	120	126	135	66+	104	106	114

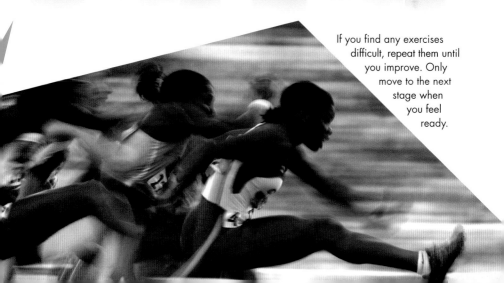

If you find any exercises difficult, repeat them until you improve. Only move to the next stage when you feel ready.

Silver workout introduction

Whether you have progressed to the Silver workout from the Bronze programme or are starting at this level, you will find that it presents new fitness challenges for your body. Some of the exercises are more advanced versions of those covered in the Bronze workout, others target different areas.

At this level, exercise intensity becomes more strenuous and it is important not to perform moves that work the same body parts consecutively. Exercises for the larger muscle groups (such as those in the legs and buttocks) should also be performed before those that challenge small muscle groups to ensure that enough oxygen is available to enable the body to perform the moves. See pages 162–3 for the suggested order of exercises.

Some of the exercises are demonstrated using water bottles as weight-training aids, but you may find that light weights are more effective for your level of strength.

The right weight for you is one that makes the last couple of repetitions of an exercise feel like hard work. In general, that will mean dumbbells weighing 1.3–2.25kg. Don't worry that weights will leave you overly muscle-bound. A woman's hormonal make-up will not predispose you to bulking up through weight training unless you devote several hours a day to lifting weights that are far heavier than those recommended in this book.

If the Silver workout seems too challenging during the first two weeks, it is worth reverting to weeks 11–12 of the Bronze workout until you can manage that with no problems. Conversely, there

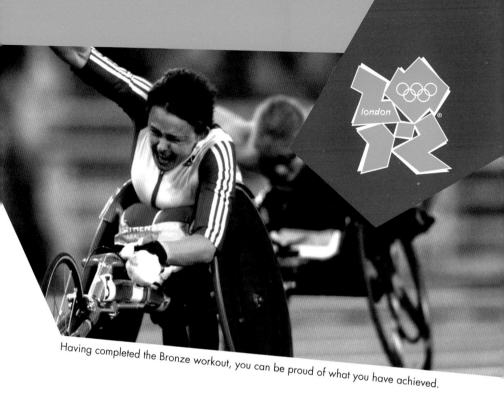

Having completed the Bronze workout, you can be proud of what you have achieved.

are more advanced alternatives to some of the moves if they seem too easy or easier versions if a particular exercise proves more challenging than others.

Silver workout schedule

Always perform a thorough warm-up and cool-down before and after a workout. Take two minutes' recovery between each set of exercises. On 2–3 other days a week, do 15–30 minutes of any aerobic activity – walking, cycling, swimming, running or indoor rowing. Try to set aside 15–30 minutes twice a week while watching television for stretching and flexibility (see pages 62–91).

Weeks	Repetitions	Weeks	Repetitions
1–2	2 sets of 8 *(of each exercise)*	7–8	3 sets of 12
3–4	2 sets of 12	9–10	2 sets of 16
5–6	3 sets of 8	11–12	4 sets of 12

Lunge

This may feel like hard work, but it's great for toning your legs and thighs.

What it does:
Strengthens the quadriceps in the front of the thigh, the hamstrings at the back of the thigh and the gluteal muscles in the buttocks.

How to do it:
1. Stand with back straight and feet hip-width apart. Bend your knees slightly making sure your hips face forward at all times. Breathe in and take a step forward with your right foot. Make sure your right foot is in line with your right knee and your left foot is raised off the ground at the heel.

Did you know?
Research conducted at the University of Wisconsin on behalf of the American Council on Exercise revealed that lunges are among the best exercises for targeting the gluteal muscles. Using electromyographic (EMG) analysis to compare the muscle activation patterns of gluteal exercises, the researchers found step-ups were as effective as squats for strengthening and toning the buttocks.

Silver workout

Too easy?

As you get stronger, drop the bent knee closer to the floor during the lunge phase. When you can manage that, have a go at the **Power lunge** in the **Gold workout** on pages 166–167.

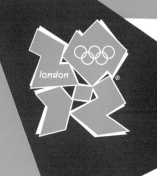

2. Lower your left knee to the ground, keeping your body weight centred over your hips throughout the movement. Lower to 15cm off the floor. Exhale and bring your right leg backwards to stand upright. Complete one set before changing legs.

Box press-up

This is an adapted version of the full press-up that will really help to tone your chest and upper body.

What it does:
Strengthens the anterior deltoids in the shoulder, the pectoral muscles in the chest and the triceps in the backs of the arms.

How to do it:
1. Kneel on all fours with your knees hip-width apart and your arms directly beneath your shoulders, fingers facing forwards. Make sure your back is flat and your head in line with your spine.

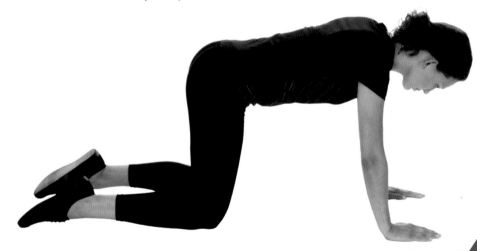

Too hard?
If you find this difficult to manage, start with the **Wall press-up** in the **Bronze workout** on pages 100–101.

Silver workout

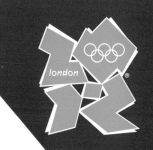

2. Breathe in as you bend your elbows and lower your upper body towards the floor. Try to touch the floor with the tip of your nose. Hold that position briefly before pressing back up to the start position with your arms. Make sure the movement is fluid and repeat in fairly quick succession.

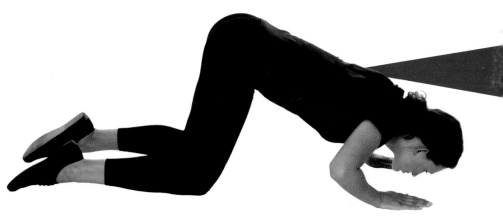

Did you know?
Stretching your neck too far forward in an effort to touch the floor is bad news as it puts strain on your neck. Use the muscles in your arms to lower yourself down without stretching the back.

Inner thigh raise

This exercise may look simple, but it really works the insides of the legs.

What it does:
Strengthens the adductor muscles in the inner thigh.

How to do it:
1. Lie on the floor on your right side with your back straight and with your head, shoulders, knees and ankles in line. Keep your abdominals pulled in. Put your left leg on the floor in front of your body for support and slightly flex your right foot. Support your head on your right hand and place your left hand on the floor in front of you.

Did you know?
Strong inner thigh muscles are essential for swimming breaststroke. Contrary to popular opinion, up to 80 per cent of the propulsion in breaststroke comes from the legs, not the arms, and this exercise will help to increase your power in the water.

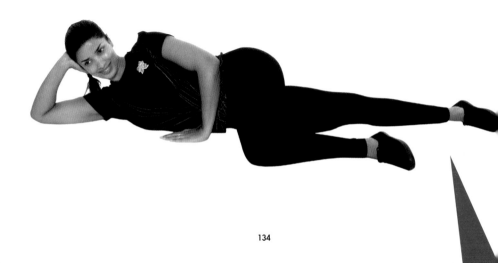

Silver workout

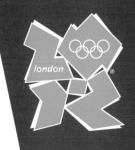

Too easy?
Once your inner thighs
are strong enough, try the
Advanced inner thigh raises in the
Gold workout on pages 188–189.

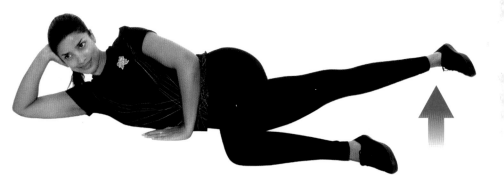

2. Slowly raise your right leg off the floor as high as
you can without wobbling off balance. Keep your left
leg stable. Hold the position for 2-4 seconds before
lowering the leg slowly back down. Perform a set on
one side before changing over.

Gluteal raise

Make sure you tense your buttock muscles during the lifting phase of this move for maximum toning effect.

What it does:
Strengthens and tones the gluteal muscles in the buttocks.

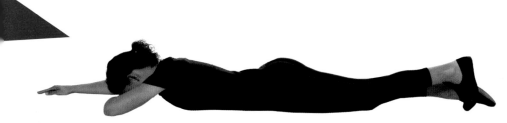

How to do it:
1. Lie face down with your hips pressed into the floor. Rest your head on your left forearm and extend your right arm in front of your body, placing the palm flat on the floor. Keep your legs straight and knees next to each other. Tense your buttock muscles and flex your left foot.

Did you know?
Studies have shown that people with weak or under-conditioned gluteal muscles are more prone to lower back pain. Strengthening the gluteal muscles with exercises like this one will help to provide stability for the lumbar region.

Silver workout

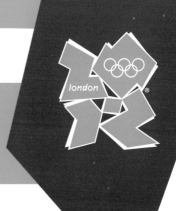

What not to do
This exercise should not cause straining in the lower back.
Stop at once if you feel pain.

Too easy?
Try the **Advanced gluteal lift** in the **Gold workout** on pages 192–193.

2. Breathe in and as you exhale raise your left foot as high off the ground as you can without arching the back or causing any discomfort. Make sure your hips remain in contact with the floor. Hold at the top of the move before lowering your leg slowly back down. Complete a full set before changing sides.

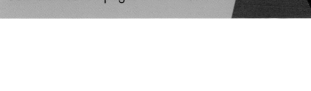

Forward raise

This exercise can be quite demanding so make sure you try the move without weights first.

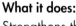

What it does:
Strengthens the anterior deltoid muscles at the front of the shoulders and the pectoral muscles in the chest.

How to do it:
1. Hold a dumbbell or a bottle of water in each hand. Stand with back straight, feet hip-width apart and abdominal muscles tucked in. Tilt your pelvis forward and bend your knees slightly. Position the weights on the front of your thighs, palms facing your body. Take a breath in.

Did you know?
You can't actually firm up the breasts' fatty tissue, but you can give the impression of improved pertness by strengthening the pectoral muscles that surround them. Push-ups and swimming breaststroke are both great bust-toners, but exercises like the Forward raise are also important.

Silver workout

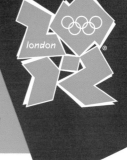

2. As you breathe out, lift the weights to shoulder height, leading with the knuckles. Keep the arms straight and level, but do not lock the elbows. Hold briefly at the top of the move before lowering the weights back down in a controlled way. Repeat.

What not to do
Don't raise the weights above shoulder height as you will strain your back.

Alternate bicep curl

This is an intensive move that can really improve tone in the upper arm.

What it does:
Strengthens the biceps muscles in the front of the arms.

How to do it:

1. Stand with feet hip-width apart and with a dumbbell or bottle of water in each hand. Bend your knees slightly and relax your arms at your sides, keeping elbows tucked in and palms facing inwards.

Tone up

Too hard?
Try the **Dumbbell curl** exercise in the **Bronze workout** on pages 96–97.

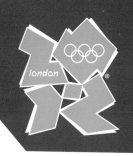

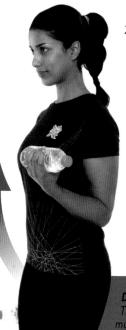

2. Breathe out and bend your left arm at the elbow to raise the weight to shoulder height. Turn the weight to the shoulder and contract your bicep muscle. Breathe in and lower the weight to the start position. Repeat on the other arm. Complete one set with alternating lifts, then repeat.

Did you know?
The function of the biceps, the major muscle in the front of the upper arm, is to provide the strength to bend the elbow and to turn the forearm so the palm of the hand faces upwards. In sport, the biceps are particularly important in throwing events such as the javelin and shot put, but also in sports that involve overhead power shots such as tennis and badminton.

Intermediate crunch

Don't rush this exercise – keep it slow and controlled for maximum firming of the stomach muscles.

What it does:
Works the rectus abdominus muscle in the abdominal areas.

How to do it:
1. Lie on your back with knees bent and feet flat on the floor, hip width apart. Press your lower back into the floor to avoid arching and contract your abdominal muscles. Keep your head level and cross your hands over your chest. Breathe in.

Don't rush

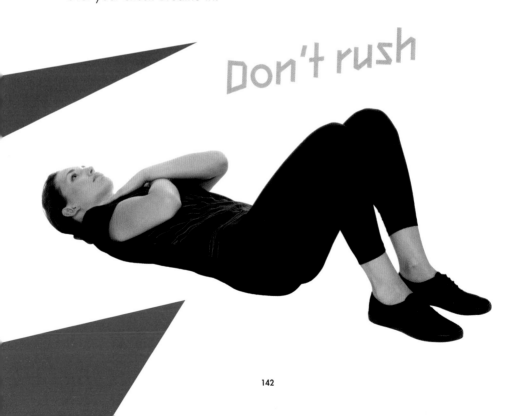

Silver workout

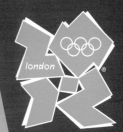

Too hard?
If you struggle with this exercise,
first master the **Beginner crunch** in
the **Bronze workout** on page 121.

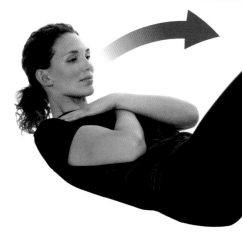

2. Exhale and slowly raise your shoulders off the floor
in a small, controlled movement, without tilting
your head forward. Do not sit up completely. Hold
the position briefly before lowering back to brush
the floor with your shoulders. Repeat.

Did you know?
*Olympic cyclists spend a lot of time developing abdominal
strength with exercises like this one. Most of the power to
pedal and stay balanced on a bike comes from the body's
core muscles that wrap around the abdominal area like a
corset. But although cycling relies on core strength, it doesn't
build it. Improving your core strength will not only improve your
fitness in everyday life, but will enhance your cycling performance.
The less energy your body needs to devote to keeping upright, the
more it can devote to pedal power.*

Reverse curl

This is a tough exercise, but one well worth doing
if you are after a toned midriff.

What it does:
Strengthens and tones the muscles in the abdominal area.

How to do it:
1. Lie on your back with legs raised in the air and
arms by your sides, palms flat on the floor. Keep
your knees slightly bent and your lower back
pressed down. Breathe in.

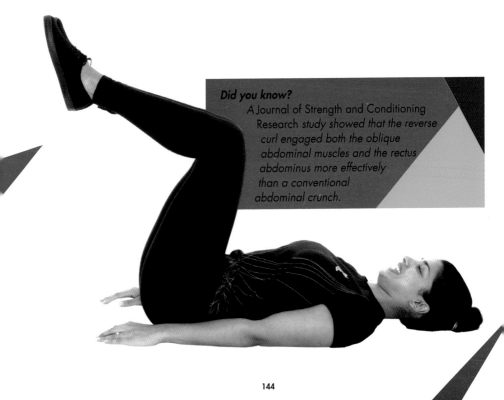

Did you know?
A Journal of Strength and Conditioning
Research *study showed that the reverse
curl engaged both the oblique
abdominal muscles and the rectus
abdominus more effectively
than a conventional
abdominal crunch.*

Silver workout

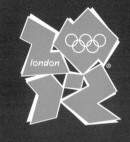

Too hard?
If you find this exercise too difficult,
try the **Beginner crunch** in the
Bronze workout on page 121.

2. Contract your abdominal muscles and
breathe out, curling your legs and pelvis
towards your chest in the process. Keep your
head and shoulders in contact with the floor
and straighten your legs until they are at a
90-degree angle to your upper body. Breathe
in and lower your legs back down to the start
position, using abdominal muscles for control.

How to make training more fun

Even the most diverse training programme can seem monotonous after a while. At such times, elite athletes struggle as much as the rest of us to get out of the door. Here are some tried and tested ways to inject the fun factor into your workouts so that boredom and tedium are erased.

Listen to music

Researchers at Brunel University showed that some exercisers who listened to music put in up to 10 per cent more effort without realising it. Not everyone benefits from listening to a good tune, though. Sport psychologists say there are two types of exerciser: associators, who are entirely tuned in to their workout, and disassociators, who like to switch off and forget what they are doing. If you fall into the former camp you may find music an unnecessary intrusion when you exercise.

Get a gadget

The market for high-tech training aids has mushroomed in recent years and while they are certainly not a necessity, gadgets – such as heart-rate monitors, pedometers and online, electronic training devices that will set and pace your training sessions, as well as provide feedback (sometimes pre-recorded from leading athletes) when you download your data to a computer after each session – can bring out your inner geek and provide a whole new dimension to your workouts.

Find a training partner

Working out with others could even be mentally soothing. Psychologists at Harvard University found that whereas a solo jog appeared to raise stress levels and stifle neurogenesis – the production of new brain cells – running with others had the opposite effect. It is thought that social interaction somehow buffers the body and brain from stressful experiences. Your training partner needn't even be human. Dogs come as a ready-made incentive for their owners to take a daily bout of exercise. Surveys have proved that dog owners are less likely to be obese, sedentary or depressed.

Add variety

Even the most dedicated and single-minded Olympians need variety to recharge interest levels in their training programme. Trying something new every week, whether it's a different exercise, a change of venue or a change of terrain – from road to trails when you run, indoors to outdoors when you cycle or incorporating hills on your daily walk – can help to keep your exercise interesting.

Join a club or class

If most of your training is done alone, joining a weekly fitness class or a local club will not only provide your workouts with an injection of sociability but also open your eyes to new techniques and training methods. Never assume that you know everything there is to know about fitness – even Olympians appreciate that the best way to learn the tricks of their trade is from those who have experimented with different training methods and pushed back the boundaries of what is possible.

Lower abdomen raise

Press your hands down during this exercise to help keep your body stable – and remember to focus on the core muscles as you raise your body.

What it does:
Strengthens and tones the lower pelvic and core muscles in the abdomen.

How to do it:
1. Lie on your back with both knees bent and feet flat on the floor, hip-width apart. Press your back into the floor and tighten your abdominal muscles. Place your hands out to your sides and breathe in.

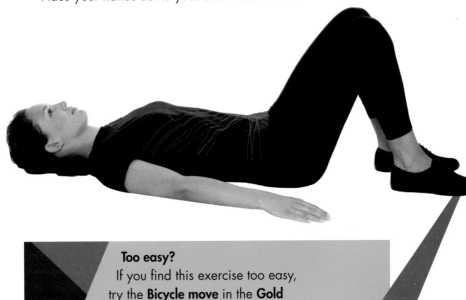

Too easy?
If you find this exercise too easy, try the **Bicycle move** in the **Gold workout** on pages 168–169.

Silver workout

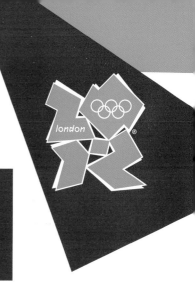

Did you know?
This exercise (also known as bridging) not only helps to improve core stability but encourages use of the gluteal muscles during activities like running, which reduces the emphasis on the quadriceps in the front of the thigh.

2. As you breathe out, lift your abdominal area, imagining you are drawing your stomach and hips up with a string. Keep your upper back on the floor. Hold briefly at the top of the move before breathing in again and lowering back down.

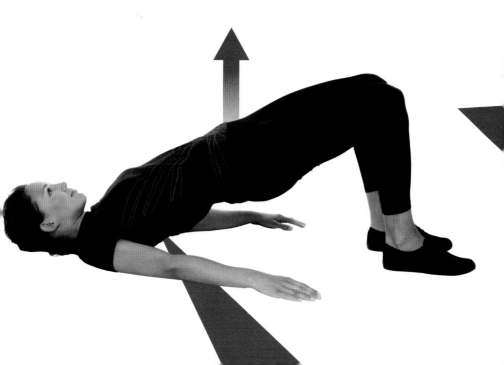

Lateral raise

This upper body exercise will help to strengthen the under-used muscles in the shoulder area.

What it does:
Works the medial deltoid muscles in the shoulders.

How to do it:
1. Stand with feet hip-width apart, back straight and abdominal muscles contracted. Tilt your pelvis forward but keep your hips square to the front. Bend your knees slightly and hold dumbbells or bottles of water in your hands at the front of your thighs.

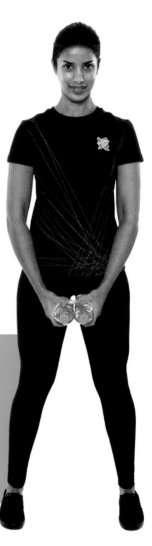

Too hard?
Make sure the weights you are using are not too heavy. Not only will it make the exercise more difficult but it can cause straining and pain in the back.

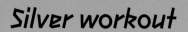

Take your time

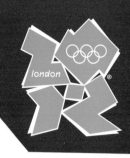

2. Breathe out as you extend your arms out to the sides in a sweeping semi-circle, leading with your knuckles. Raise the weights to shoulder-height without locking your elbows. Turn your wrists upwards so that your knuckles face the ceiling. Keep the weights parallel to the floor. Hold briefly before breathing in and lowering the weights back to the start position. Repeat.

Bench step-up

This simple exercise is among the most effective leg and bottom strengthening moves around.

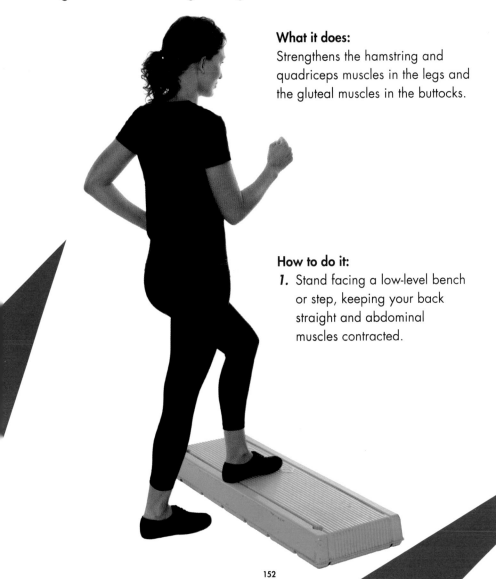

What it does:
Strengthens the hamstring and quadriceps muscles in the legs and the gluteal muscles in the buttocks.

How to do it:
1. Stand facing a low-level bench or step, keeping your back straight and abdominal muscles contracted.

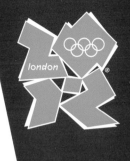

step up

2. Step up onto the bench with the whole of your right foot, then the whole of your left foot. Step back down, right foot first, then left foot. Breathe evenly throughout the exercise.

Reverse Fly

Remember not to bend or curve your back when you perform this exercise – keep your shoulders relaxed.

What it does:
Works the posterior deltoid muscles in the upper back and the muscles in the shoulders.

How to do it:
1. Stand with feet hip-width apart and knees slightly bent. Lean forward from your hips, keeping your back straight. Hold bottles of water or weights in each hand and extend your arms down in front of you.

Did you know?
The reverse fly is widely used by rowers, who need strong back muscles to pull through each stroke. But physiotherapists consider the exercise to be important in creating good muscular balance in many other sports – particularly those that involve throwing – because it targets muscles that are often underused.

Relax

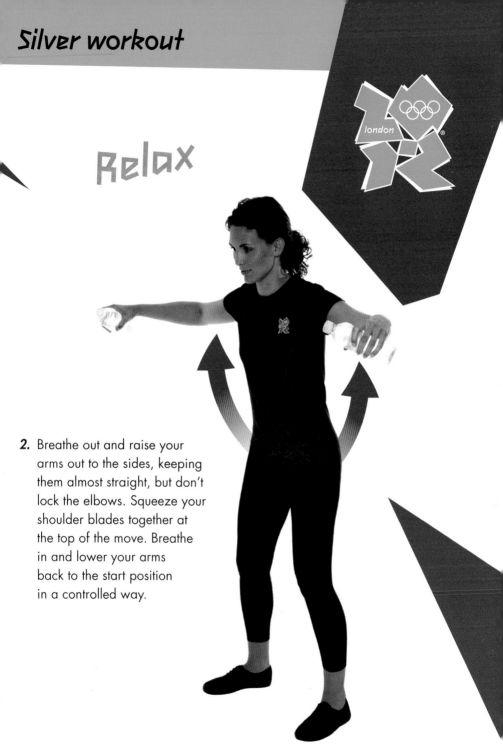

2. Breathe out and raise your arms out to the sides, keeping them almost straight, but don't lock the elbows. Squeeze your shoulder blades together at the top of the move. Breathe in and lower your arms back to the start position in a controlled way.

Intermediate lower back raise

Perform this exercise regularly and it will help to improve your posture and breathing efficiency.

What it does:
Works the erector spinae muscles in the lower back.

How to do it:
1. Lie on the floor face down with legs extended and toes pointing downwards. Place your hands beneath your chin and keep your head in line with your spine. Breathe in.

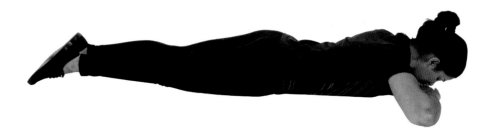

Did you know?
The erector spinae is a collection of three muscles running along your neck to your lower back. They work together with the core muscles to support the back and provide good posture, which is vital in sport for preventing injury.

Silver workout

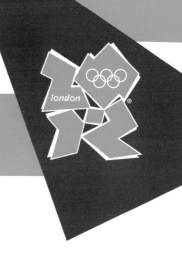

Too hard?
Try the **Beginner lower back raise** in
the **Bronze workout** on pages 102–103.

Enjoy the workout

2. As you breathe out, raise your upper body off the
floor in a smooth and controlled movement. Keep your
hips pressed down and hold the position at the top of
the movement. Breathe in and slowly lower the upper
body back down. Repeat.

Single leg squat

This move can be trickier to master than some, but it is well worth the effort if you want strong legs and thighs.

What it does:
Strengthens the hamstring muscles in the backs of the legs and the gluteal muscles in the buttocks.

How to do it:
1. Stand with feet hip-width apart and arms extended to the front (or to the sides if you find this easier).

Too hard?
If you find this exercise too difficult, try the **Seated squat** in the **Bronze workout** on pages 112–113.

2. Take your left foot off the floor and slowly lower your bottom backwards as if you are going to sit down. Allow your upper body to lean forward slightly as you lower your bottom, but make sure your back remains straight. Try not to wobble – make sure the knee bends directly over the right foot. To make the exercise harder, extend your left leg in front of you at the lowest squat point.

Strength and balance

Did you know?
In tests at the physiology and biomechanics laboratories of the University of Wisconsin, the single leg squat out-performed seated squats in terms of working the gluteal medius muscle in the buttocks. It also worked the hamstring and gluteus maximus muscles harder than the vertical leg press machine at the gym.

Single arm row

Great for toning the upper back and the triceps and biceps muscles in the upper arm.

What it does:
Strengthens the latissimus dorsi muscles in the mid-back, deltoids in the shoulders and the biceps in the backs of the arms.

Did you know?
This exercise is particularly useful for runners and sprinters as it boosts power in the muscles involved in a strong arm action, improving the ability to pull back the elbow in a straight, efficient line alongside the body.

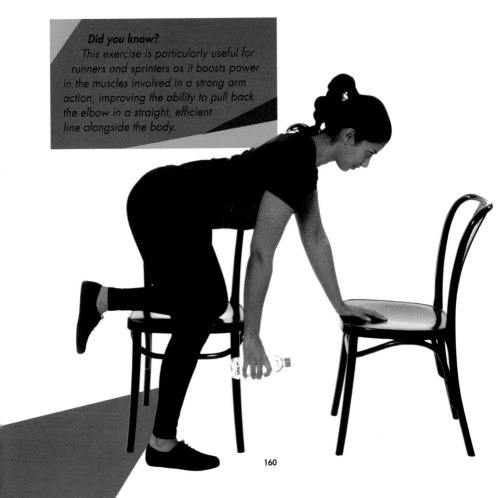

Silver workout

How to do it:

1. Stand sideways on – left side nearest – to a bench or chair, holding a dumbbell in your right hand. Bend your left knee and place it on the bench. Support yourself with your left hand on the bench, slightly in front of your left shoulder. Keep the elbow slightly flexed. Bend your right knee slightly, but keep your foot flat on the floor. Allow the right hand to fall straight down as it holds the dumbbell. Make sure your back is straight and your head in line with your spine. Breathe in.

2. Exhale and pull the dumbbell up towards your chest in a controlled movement, keeping your elbow close to your body. Hold briefly at the top of the movement. Breathe in and lower back down. Complete a set with your right arm and then a set with your left.

Silver workout
— summary

Progression is key to any workout programme. Your muscles, cardiovascular system and even your mind thrive on being pushed to new limits. Failing to progress in an exercise routine means not only that your fitness levels will stall, but also that you will get bored and be more likely to quit.

As you tackle more challenging and intense workouts, you may notice that your body responds in unfamiliar ways. If you wake up the morning after an exercise session feeling muscle soreness and stiffness as you reach over to turn off the alarm, it is likely that you are experiencing Delayed Onset Muscle Soreness (DOMS). Unlike immediate muscle soreness – the kind you experience during and straight after a workout and which quickly dissipates – DOMS can arise anything between 24–48 hours after you finish and persist for up to 72 hours following your session.

Do not think that DOMS is a sign of a lack of fitness – on the contrary, even Olympic athletes experience it, often taking it as a rewarding sign that they are working hard enough. But it can also affect newcomers to activity or those who have stepped up their activity levels.

Making progress

What causes DOMS and what can you do about it?

As much as it may feel slightly uncomfortable, DOMS is a positive sign that your body is adapting to intense activity. Nobody knows precisely what causes it, but most studies suggest that it is the result of microscopic tears in connective tissue surrounding muscles after a hard workout involving eccentric muscle contractions. Muscles contract eccentrically whenever they lengthen under tension. That can mean during a dumbbell curl, when the biceps in the front of the arm lengthen and shorten during the lifting and lowering, but also when you run downhill the quadriceps in the front of the thigh lengthen and shorten in response to gravity. Researchers have yet to prove that anything significantly hastens recovery from DOMS, although there is some evidence that applying ice (or having a cool bath), massage and stretching can help. The good news is that once you have experienced DOMS after a few sessions at a new level, you are unlikely to have it again until you increase the duration and intensity once more.

Suggested order of exercises

As with the other workout plans in this book, the order in which the exercises are done is not entirely prescriptive. However, it is best not to perform consecutive exercises on the same muscle groups. Here is a suggested order of action:

- Lunge *(pages 130–131)*
- Box press-up *(pages 132–133)*
- Inner thigh raise *(pages 134–135)*
- Alternate bicep curl *(pages140–141)*
- Intermediate crunch *(pages 142–143)*
- Gluteal raise *(pages 136–137)*
- Lateral raise *(pages 150–151)*
- Lower abdomen raise *(pages 148–149)*
- Bench step up *(pages 152–153)*
- Reverse fly *(pages154–155)*
- Single leg squat *(pages 158–159)*
- Forward raise *(pages 138–139)*
- Intermediate lower back raise *(pages 156–157)*
- Reverse curl *(pages 144–145)*
- Single arm row *(pages 160–161)*

Gold workout introduction

Welcome to the top of the rostrum in terms of the training programmes outlined in this book. The Gold workout may not win you an Olympic medal of the same colour, but it will provide the springboard to propel you to a competitive level of fitness.

If you have progressed through the Bronze and Silver programmes in this book, you will notice that the number of repetitions and exercises in this section are greater, making the Gold workout not only more challenging in terms of the effort required, but more time-consuming. Although this will ultimately pay dividends, the extra work involved can sometimes cause a fitness plateau, a point at which improvements level off.

If this happens, listen to your body and take stock of the work you have been doing. It could be that you need to schedule in more rest to your lifestyle or that you are lifting weights that are too heavy or too light to make improvements. Or

maybe it is your mind that is weary of working out and not your body? Injecting variety and fun into your workout (see pages 146–147 for tips on how to do this) can help you to rekindle your enjoyment and start to reap the benefits from the effort you are making again. The key is not to get disheartened or disillusioned. Simple tweaks to your routine can make exercise enjoyable and rewarding again.

As in the Silver workout, the exercises in this programme are intense and should not be performed on the same body parts consecutively. See pages 196–197 for a suggested order. Remember that in exercises that require the use of weights, the weight

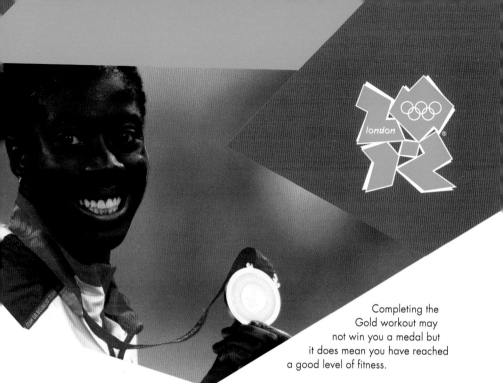

Completing the Gold workout may not win you a medal but it does mean you have reached a good level of fitness.

you lift should be sufficiently heavy to make the last few repetitions in each set feel like hard work, but not so heavy that they are impossible to perform. At this level, you may find dumbbells of anything from 1.3 to 3kg appropriate.

Gold workout schedule

Always perform a thorough warm up and cool down before and after a workout. Take two minutes recovery between each set of exercises. On 2–3 other days a week, do 20–40 minutes of any aerobic activity – walking, cycling, swimming, running or indoor rowing. Try to set aside 15–30 minutes twice a week while watching television for stretching and flexibility (see pages 62–91).

Weeks	Repetitions	Weeks	Repetitions
1–2	3 sets of 8 *(of each exercise)*	7–8	4 sets of 12
3–4	3 sets of 12	9–10	3 sets of 16
5–6	4 sets of 8	11–12	4 sets of 16

Power lunge

The perfect exercise for toning the legs and buttocks, this is a staple of all exercise programmes.

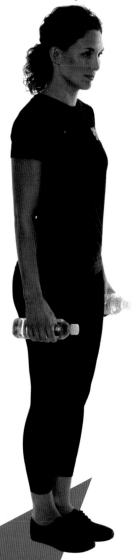

What it does:
Strengthens the quadriceps in the front of the thigh, the hamstrings at the back of the thigh and the gluteal muscles in the buttocks.

How to do it:
1. Stand with your back straight and feet hip-width apart, holding bottles of water or weights in each hand. Bend your knees slightly, making sure your hips face forward at all times. Breathe in and take a step forward with your left foot. Make sure your left foot is in line with your left knee and your right foot raised off the ground at the heel.

Did you know?
Lunges are a favourite exercise of Olympic sprinters and footballers because of their ability to boost leg strength in muscles that provide the power to run faster. A six-week study in which footballers performed lunges twice a week as part of their training showed marked improvements in hamstring strength and a decrease in muscle pain during exercise.

Gold workout

Too hard?
If you find this exercise too difficult, first try the **Lunge** in the **Silver workout** on pages 130–131.

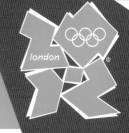

2. Lower your right knee to within 5cm of the ground, keeping your body weight centred over your hips throughout the movement. Exhale and bring your right leg backwards to stand upright. Complete one set before changing legs.

Bicycle move

The bicycle move gets a gold-star rating from the experts, who say it is great for toning the midriff.

What it does:
Strengthens the rectus abdominus and the external oblique muscles in the abdominal area.

How to do it:
1. Lie on your back with knees bent and feet flat on the floor. Press your lower back into the floor, engaging your abdominal muscles, as you put both hands lightly behind your head (don't pull).

Too hard?
To make it easier, keep your knees bent and tap your feet to the floor rather than extending your leg straight out.

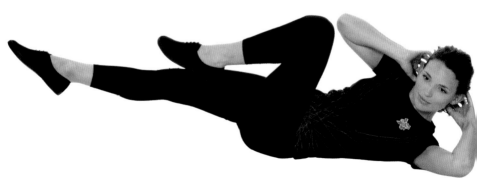

Gold workout

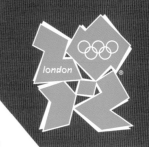

2. Bring your right elbow over to your left knee, then your left elbow over to your right knee in alternate twisting moves while pedalling your legs. Breathe steadily. Turn each elbow towards the opposite knee, with hands held lightly behind your head, in a slow, controlled way, with full extension of each leg on all repetitions.

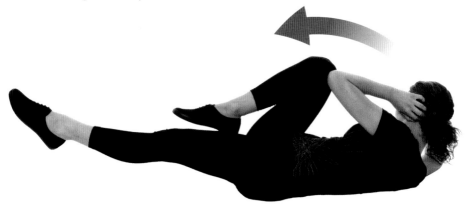

Did you know?
A study at San Diego State University looked at 13 of the most popular abdomen-strengthening exercises, ranking them best to worst. Using specialist electromyography equipment, researchers recorded muscle activity in the upper and lower rectus abdominus and in the external oblique muscles. Among the most effective was the Bicycle move, which used 290 per cent more muscle energy than a conventional crunch exercise.

Advanced crunch

An exercise included in the training regimes of most sprinters and power-based athletes.

What it does:
Works all the major muscles in the abdominal area, including the rectus abdominus and external obliques.

How to do it:

1. Lie on your back with feet raised off the floor and knees bent at a 90-degree angle. Cup your hands lightly at the sides of your head and contract your abdominal muscles.

Did you know?
Strong abdominal muscles are crucial in any sport that involves twisting motions from around the trunk – taekwondo, wrestling, boxing, canoe slalom and sprint are just a few examples.

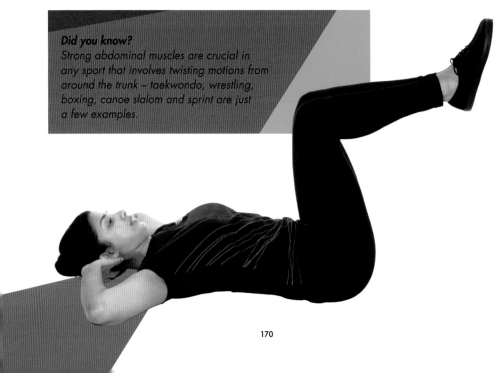

Gold workout

Too hard?
Try the **Beginner crunch** in the **Bronze workout** on page 121 or the **Intermediate crunch** in the **Silver workout** on pages 142–143 before progressing to this demanding move.

2. Lift your shoulder blades off the floor and curl them forwards towards your knees in a small, controlled movement. Don't bring your knees towards your chest. Keep your lower back pressed down to prevent arching and keep your chin raised. Breathe in and lower back down, allowing your shoulders to brush the floor before repeating the move.

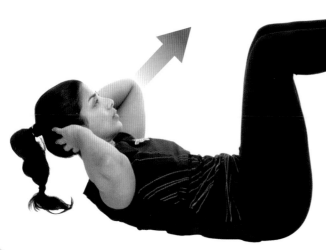

Full press-up

The press-up is renowned for being the best all-over conditioning move around.

What it does:
Strengthens the pectoral muscles in the chest, triceps in the backs of the arms, anterior deltoids in the shoulders, the core abdominal muscles, hamstring and quadriceps muscles in the thighs.

How to do it:

1. Lie face down with feet hip-width apart and hands at shoulder height, about 30–35cm from your body. Your fingertips should be pointing forwards. Press up onto your toes, keeping your back flat and abdominal muscles contracted. Your head should be in line with your spine.

Top tip
To work the shoulder muscles more intensively, position your hands closer to your body. The further out you move your hands, the harder you will be working the muscles in the chest.

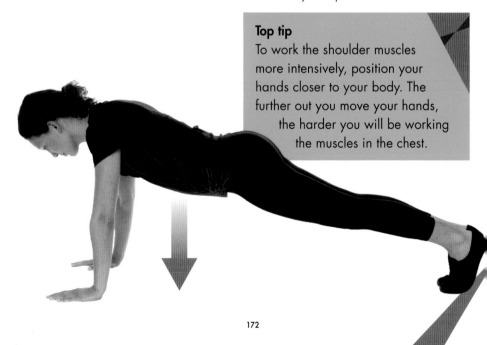

Gold workout

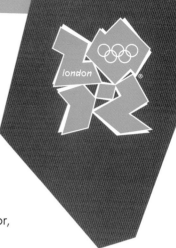

Do your best

2. Breathe in and lower your body towards the floor, aiming to touch it with your chest, but do not lie down. Hold briefly before pressing back up using your arms. Do not allow the elbows to lock at the top of the move. Repeat in a fluid motion.

Did you know?
Why the popularity of the press-up has endured among top athletes becomes clear when you learn how many muscles it tests – those in the arms, chest, abdomen and legs – with each repetition. Researchers in one US trial showed that, on average, 66.4 per cent of total body weight is lifted with each push-up. So if you weigh 70kg you are heaving a mighty 46kg – far more than you would on a bench-press machine.

Tricep dip

The perfect move for reducing flab that hangs at the backs of the arms.

What it does:
Strengthens the triceps muscles in the backs of the arms.

How to do it:
1. Sit on a chair and shift yourself forward until your bottom is on the edge of the seat. Place hands on the edge of the chair for support and move your bottom off the chair, taking the weight in your arms and hands. Keep your back straight and head in line with your spine. Extend your legs in front of you and bend your knees so that they are at right angles.

Gold workout

Safety notes
- Always make sure the room you are using is well-ventilated when you work out.
- Don't perform exercises on a slippery floor surface or on a rug/mat that might move when you step on it.
- Make sure there is plenty of room to move upwards, backwards and sideways.
- Make sure that all equipment you are using (such as chairs and benches) is stable and can bear your weight before you attempt the relevant exercise.

2. Keep your feet flat on the floor and breathe in as you slowly lower the body in a straight line towards the floor. Dip down as low as your strength will allow, hold the low position briefly and then push back up using your arms (not your legs) to the start position. Repeat.

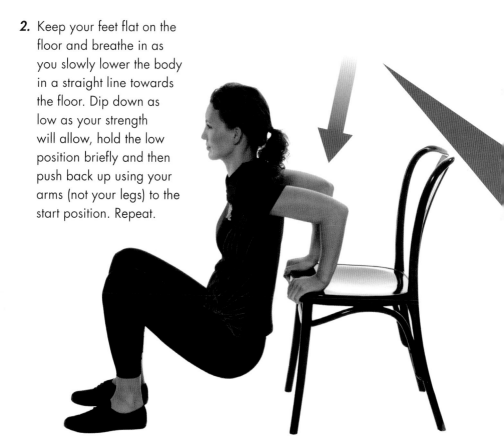

Plié squat

Squats are great for firming the buttocks and thighs, and this advanced version will really improve strength and tone in those areas.

What it does:
Works the quadriceps, hamstring and gluteal muscles in the thighs and buttocks.

How to do it:
1. Hold one dumbbell or a bottle of water with both hands at the centre of your body. Place your feet wider than shoulder-width apart and turn your toes out to an angle of 45 degrees. Keep your back straight, head lifted and in line with the spine and your abdominal muscles tucked in.

Too hard?
If you find this move too difficult, try mastering it without the weights. Place your hands on your hips as you squat or use the back of a dining chair for support.

Gold workout

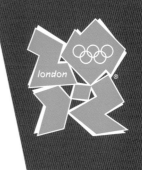

2. Relax your shoulders and breathe in as you bend with the knees and hips in a plié position, keeping the weight close to your body. Keep your knees in line with your feet to ensure that you are well balanced. Breathe out and slowly return to the standing position, keeping your heels fixed to the floor.

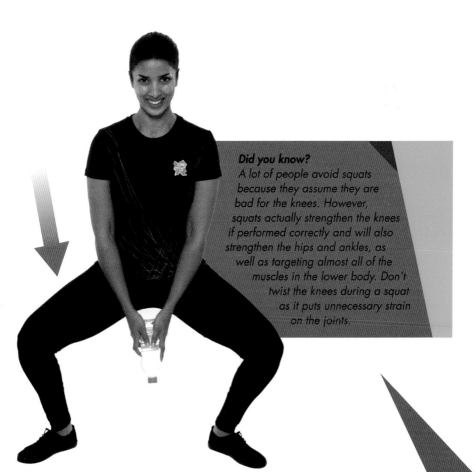

Did you know?
A lot of people avoid squats because they assume they are bad for the knees. However, squats actually strengthen the knees if performed correctly and will also strengthen the hips and ankles, as well as targeting almost all of the muscles in the lower body. Don't twist the knees during a squat as it puts unnecessary strain on the joints.

The plank

Supporting your own body weight with exercises like the plank is among the best ways to build strength.

What it does:
Strengthens the rectus abdominus and transversus abdominus in the trunk as well as muscles in the lower back.

How to do it:

1. Lie face down on the floor, resting on the forearms, with palms flat on the ground at shoulder height.

Did you know?
Top rowers and canoeists rely on good core stability to allow them to apply power correctly during every stroke. Studies at the San Diego State University found the plank exercise to be among the most effective abdomen-strengthening moves around.

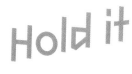

Hold it

Gold workout

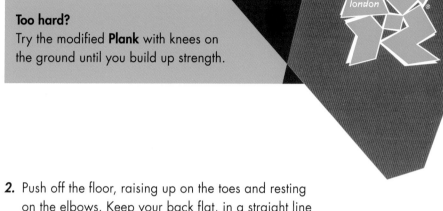

Too hard?
Try the modified **Plank** with knees on
the ground until you build up strength.

2. Push off the floor, raising up on the toes and resting
on the elbows. Keep your back flat, in a straight line
from head to heels. Tilt your pelvis and contract your
abdominal muscles to prevent your bottom from sticking
up or sagging. Hold the position for 15–20 seconds.

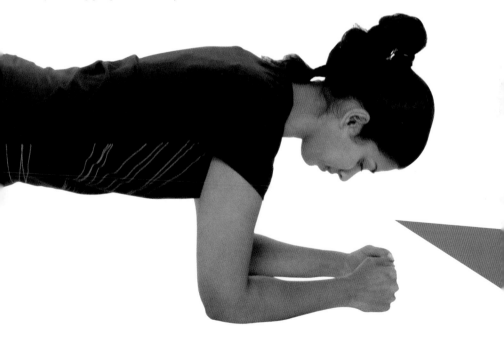

How to get the Olympic edge

In pursuit of Olympic success, athletes and their coaches are forever pushing back the boundaries of fitness and training. Here are some of the methods they use to help them get that Olympic edge.

Training your inspiratory muscles

Hand-held respiratory training devices that strengthen the muscles used to breathe are widely used by cyclists, rowers, runners and swimmers. Research at Indiana University showed that six weeks of inspiratory muscle training reduced the amount of oxygen required during exercise, making more oxygen available for muscles elsewhere in the body.

Getting enough sleep

The English Institute of Sport's performance laboratories studied the effects of sleep on the performance levels of 60 elite athletes. Their findings suggest that adequate rest affects not only performance but recovery from vigorous physical activity. Missing sleep for a couple of nights is unlikely to have much impact on your gym performance – many champions get little sleep the night before an Olympic final – but chronic sleep deprivation will almost certainly take its toll. Scientists who analysed the sleep/wake patterns of five sporty females who were getting between six and eight hours sleep a night found they were able to run faster, hit tennis balls more accurately and exhibit greater arm strength when they extended their sleeping hours to 10.

Cool it

At the Athens 2004 and Beijing 2008 Olympic Games, many British athletes prepared for the searing temperatures by wearing a pre-cool vest that discreetly holds ice packs in its lining to reduce core body temperature by 19 per cent and minimise heat injury and dehydration risk. But there is a simpler way to help your body to prepare for exercise in warm weather: drink a slushy ice drink before you head out. In a study, athletes who drank a syrup-flavoured ice drink just before running on a treadmill in a hot room could keep going for an average of 50 minutes before they had to stop. When they drank only syrup-flavoured cold water, they could run for an average of 40 minutes.

Sports drinks

Just a 2 per cent drop in hydration levels can severely limit athletic performance, so the replacement of lost fluid and electrolytes (body salts) is a priority for athletes. Prior to each Games, experts at the British Olympic Medical Institute formulate a sports drink to meet the precise hydration needs of athletes, altering the formula according to the temperature and humidity in the country where the Games are to be held. For the rest of us, sports drinks are not necessary in non-intense activities lasting less than an hour. But if you are training hard or preparing for an endurance event, then an isotonic drink containing tiny particles of easily digestible carbohydrates can enhance fluid uptake and top up the body's stores of glycogen, its preferred source of fuel.

Advanced calf raise

Strong calf muscles are important for most sports, but also for everyday activities like walking and jogging.

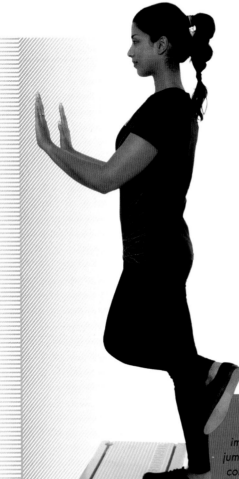

What it does:
Strengthens the muscles in the calf.

How to do it:
1. Stand on a small platform, step or block of wood positioned about 30–50cm from a wall. Allow your heels to hang off the raised surface and support yourself by placing your hands on the wall at chest height, fingertips facing upwards. Keep your back straight and put your right foot behind your left calf just above the ankle.

Did you know?
Strength in the calf muscles is very important for improvements in speed and jump height, which are critical athletic components in the high jump, long jump and triple jump events as well as in volleyball and gymnastics.

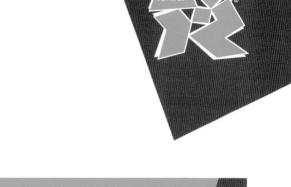

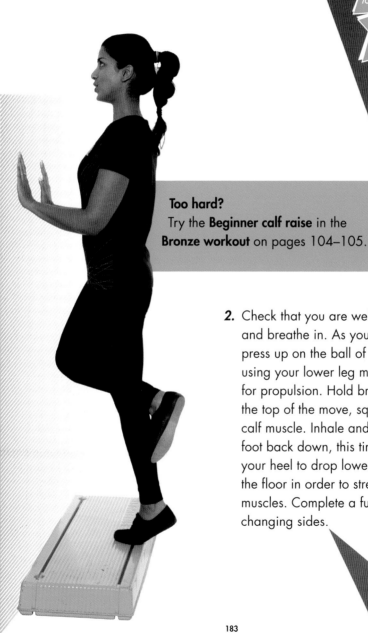

Too hard?
Try the **Beginner calf raise** in the **Bronze workout** on pages 104–105.

2. Check that you are well balanced and breathe in. As you exhale, press up on the ball of your left foot using your lower leg muscles for propulsion. Hold briefly at the top of the move, squeezing your calf muscle. Inhale and lower your foot back down, this time allowing your heel to drop lower towards the floor in order to stretch the muscles. Complete a full set before changing sides.

Advanced leg extension

Great for improving the shape and tone of the upper leg muscles.

What it does:
Strengthens the quadriceps and hamstring muscles in the thighs.

How to do it:
1. Lie back, propping yourself up on your elbows but keeping your forearms flat on the floor. Keep your back straight and head looking forward. With your feet hip-width apart and knees bent at a 90-degree angle, place your left foot flat on the floor and flex your right foot at the ankle. Breathe out and lift your right leg, keeping your knees parallel.

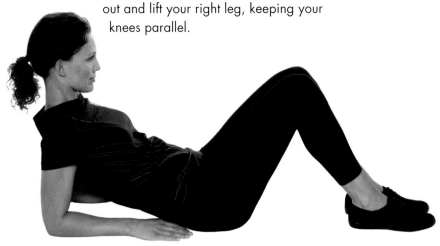

Too hard?
Try the **Beginner leg extension** in the **Bronze workout** on pages 116–117.

Gold workout

Kick on

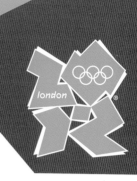

2. Hold briefly without locking your knee. Breathe
in and lower your leg back down, stopping
about 5cm from the floor. Hold briefly before
raising the leg again, leading with the foot.
Complete a set before changing sides.

Advanced hamstring curl

This exercise is perfect for adding tone to the buttocks.

What it does:
Works the hamstring and gluteus maximus muscles in the thighs and buttocks.

How to do it:
1. Kneel on all fours with legs hip-width apart, back flat and head in line with the spine. Keep your arms directly beneath your shoulders and your hands flat on the floor with fingertips facing forwards. Breathe in and extend your left leg behind you until it is parallel to the floor. Flex your foot so that the toes are pointing downwards and keep your hips square to the ground.

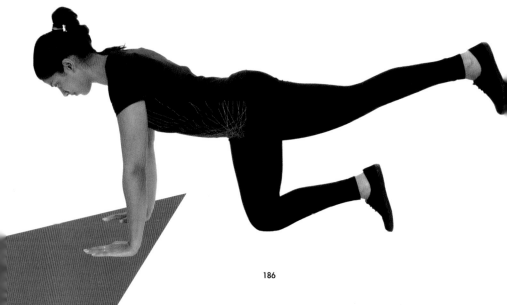

Gold workout

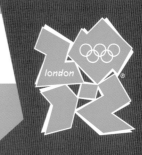

Too hard?
Try the **Beginner hamstring curl** in
the **Bronze workout** on page 120.

2. Breathe out and curl your extended left foot upwards
towards your buttocks. Hold briefly at the top of the
move. Breathe in and straighten your leg again, flexing
the foot. Complete a full set before changing sides.

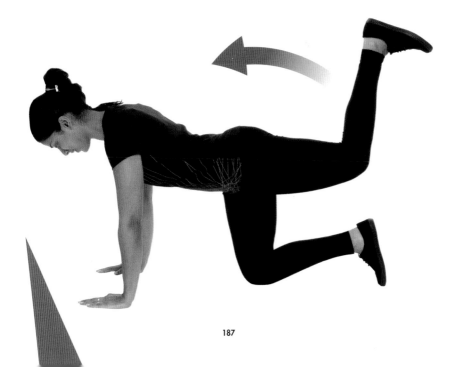

Advanced inner thigh raise

This exercise targets muscles that are often overlooked in exercise regimes.

What it does:
Strengthens the adductor muscles in the inner thigh.

How to do it:
1. Lie on your left side with your left leg extended and foot flexed. Place your right leg on the floor in front of you for stability and support your upper body by propping yourself up on your left elbow and placing your right hand on the floor in front of you. Breathe in.

Enjoy it

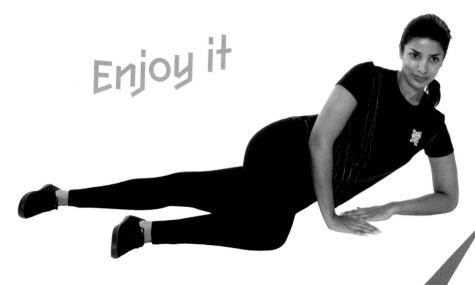

Gold workout

2. Exhale and slowly raise your left leg as high as you can, keeping your foot flexed and your leg straight. Hold at about 5–8cm off the floor before lowering back down. Complete a set on the left leg before changing sides.

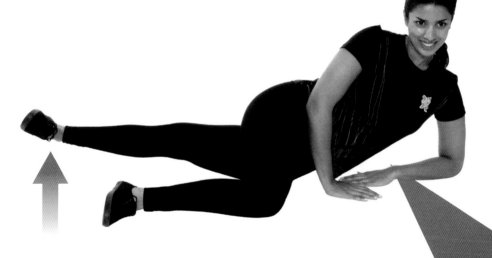

Did you know?
Strong adductor muscles are vital in sports like hockey and football as the muscles come under immense strain during sudden turning. In football they are also engaged when the ball is kicked.

Outer thigh lift

A move that will help to reduce the appearance of 'saddlebags' on the thighs.

What it does:
Strengthens and tones the abductor muscles on the outer thigh and the adductor muscles on the inner thigh.

How to do it:
1. Stand sideways to a wall with your right side nearest – you should be about 60cm away from the wall. Place your right hand on the wall at shoulder height for support and put your left hand on your hip. Keep your head facing forward and your back straight. Breathe in.

Gold workout

Too hard?
If you find this exercise too difficult, try the **Leg raise** in the **Bronze workout** on pages 108–109.

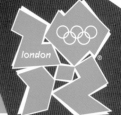

2. Slowly raise your left leg, making sure you stay upright. Don't raise it too high as you may start to lean forward. Hold briefly at the top of the move before lowering the foot back down in a slow, controlled manner. Do not let the foot return to the start position. When the foot is 2cm from the ground, lift it upwards again. Complete a set before changing sides.

Advanced gluteal lift

Strong gluteal muscles can have huge benefits in sports such as running, where they add power to every stride.

What it does:
Strengthens the gluteal muscles in the buttocks.

How to do it:
1. Kneel on all fours with knees hip-width apart. Place your arms directly beneath the shoulders with your palms flat on the floor. Keep your back flat and hips square to the floor, with your head in line with the spine. Extend your right leg out behind you, keeping the foot flexed. Breathe in.

Too hard?
Try the **Gluteal raise** in the **Silver workout** on pages 136–137.

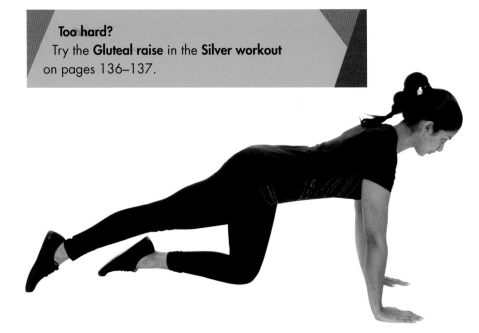

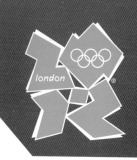

Feel the
benefits

2. Breathe out as you lift your extended leg to hip height
with the foot flexed. Hold briefly at the top of the move
before lowering down. Allow your toes to brush the
floor before repeating the move. Complete a set on
one leg before changing sides.

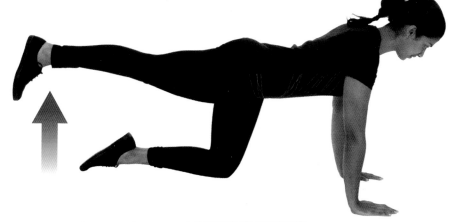

Did you know?
Once your gluteal muscles are stronger,
you could try adding some ankle weights
to increase the resistance in this exercise.
However, make sure you start with very light
weights. Trying to lift a weight that is too heavy
will cause strain in the lower back.

Bench pec fly

Breast tissue cannot be toned itself, but strong pectoral muscles in the chest help to improve breast appearance and pertness.

What it does:
Strengthens the pectoral muscles in the chest and the anterior deltoid muscles in the shoulders, as well as the biceps muscles in the front of the arms.

How to do it:
1. Lie on the floor (or on an exercise bench with feet hip-width apart and flat on the floor), holding a set of dumbbells or bottles of water in each hand. Contract your abdominal muscles and keep your head in line with your spine. Lift weights directly above you with arms outstretched.

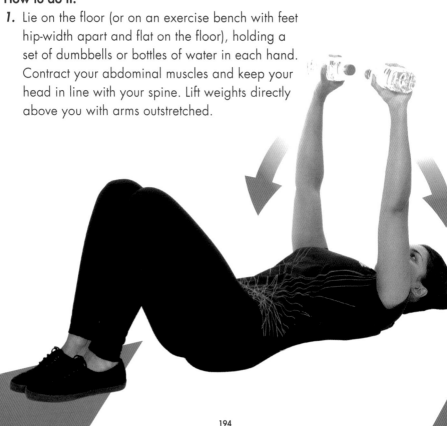

Gold workout

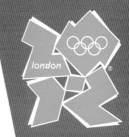

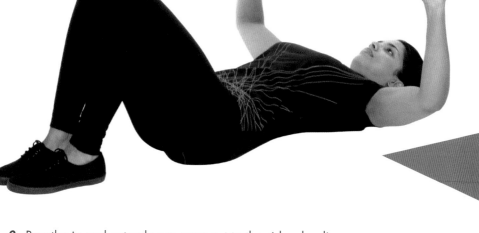

2. Breathe in and extend your arms out to the sides, leading with your elbows. Your elbows should be bent, palms facing upwards and wrists kept in line with the forearms. As you lift make sure your arms are in line with the shoulders. Stop when the weights reach shoulder or chest level. Hold the position briefly before breathing out and pressing your arms back together above your chest. Repeat.

Gold workout — summary

At this level there is much more scope to vary the way you structure your training sessions. Since you will be performing more repetitions than in the Bronze and Silver programmes, your workouts will take longer. If time is an issue, then consider splitting the routine so you perform exercises for the same body part on alternate days. Be creative and experiment to see what works for you.

Suggested order of exercises
If you do wish to perform the Gold workout in its entirety, follow the suggested order below:

- Power lunge (pages 166–167)
- Tricep dip (pages 174–175)
- Bicycle move (pages 168–169)
- Advanced calf raise
    (pages 182–183)
- Plié squat (pages 176–177)
- The plank (pages 178–179)
- Advanced leg extension
    (pages 184–185)
- Bench pec fly (pages 194–195)
- Advanced hamstring curl
    (pages 186–187)
- Outer thigh lift (pages 190–191)
- Advanced crunch
    (pages 170–171)
- Full press-up (pages 172–173)
- Advanced gluteal lift
    (pages 194–195)
- Advanced inner thigh raise
    (pages 188–189)

Increase your training zone

In some of your sessions, start to push the intensity of your exertion to 80–85% of your MHR (see page 127 in the Bronze workout for an explanation). This is a level at which you are breathing heavily and will struggle to hold a conversation. In terms of beats per minute, 80–85% MHR is as follows:

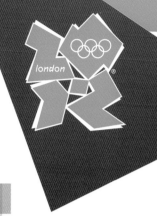

Age	MHR	Age	MHR
18–25	159–169	43–50	148–147
26–30	153–163	51–58	133–141
31–36	149–158	59–65	126–134
37–42	144–153	66+	121–129

Ways to work harder:

- If you run on a treadmill, always keep the belt at a 1 per cent incline to simulate the undulations and changes in terrain you experience outdoors.
- On walks, runs and cycles add more hills to your route. Hill training forces the body to work against gravity and is like a natural form of weight training for the legs and buttocks.
- Fartlek – the Swedish for 'speed play' – is an approach widely used by athletes in endurance sessions. It involves varying the speed between pre-determined markers (such as lamp posts or trees) on a run, cycle or power walk. Try to include as many different speeds as you can from slow and steady to flat-out sprinting.
- Skipping is a great form of exercise used by many boxers and athletes. Start with 5–10 minutes of skipping and progress until you can manage 20 minutes.

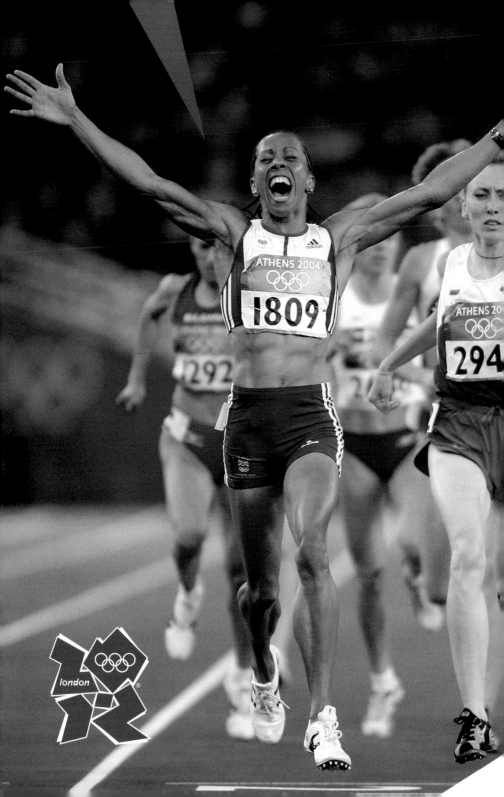

The practicalities

Regular exercise is crucial for improving your fitness, but how do you make sure that it remains part of your lifestyle? Learning how to deal with setbacks, such as illness or injury, what to eat to support your activity levels and how to boost your motivation when enthusiasm is flagging are key to long-term success.

Olympic athletes need to stay in top condition in order to compete and win. They are careful to avoid illness and injury and to eat a healthy, specially balanced diet.

Staying fit and healthy

A vital aspect of any training programme is keeping things on an even keel. Olympic athletes, together with their coaches, scrutinise every aspect of their lifestyle to make sure they are doing their utmost to avoid injury, illness and other barriers to consistent training. But it is just as important for anyone looking to improve their fitness to take precautions and steps ensure that they stay in tip-top condition.

DON'T OVERDO IT: Progression in workouts is a good thing, but push yourself too far, too soon and you could be asking for trouble. Over-training syndrome occurs when the body isn't allowed enough time to recover from the rigours of tough training sessions. There are warning signs other than soreness and fatigue that may indicate your body is suffering from chronic over-exertion. Disturbed sleep patterns, depression and mood swings, stomach problems and a raised resting heart rate all indicate that you are overdoing things on the exercise front. Take things gradually and don't perform tough sessions on consecutive days.

Stick to the 10 per cent rule, which means don't increase your usual activity by more than 10 per cent at a time.

WHEN TO STOP: You are sneezing, spluttering and have a blocked nose, so should you stop working out? A useful tip is to apply the 'below the neck' rule when you are unsure if your symptoms are severe enough to curtail your exercise routine. If you have fever, sore muscles or joints, vomiting or a very productive cough – symptoms that exhibit themselves from the neck down – then you probably need to avoid exercise for at least a couple of days. If you just have a runny or blocked nose, watery eyes and a light, tickly

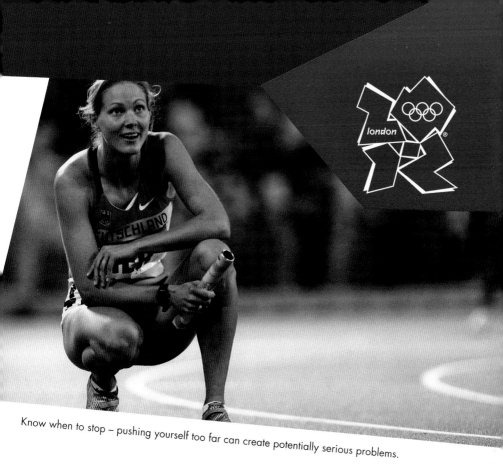

Know when to stop – pushing yourself too far can create potentially serious problems.

cough, it's generally fine to continue. Studies have shown that colds have little effect on athletic performance and that exercise doesn't aggravate symptoms such as a blocked nose and streaming eyes.

RICE IT: Because of the demands they place on their bodies, active people are more at risk of sustaining injuries. Understanding your body's strengths and weaknesses and taking precautions, such as thorough warm-ups and cool-downs and regular

stretching, can help to keep problems at bay, but if you are unlucky enough to suffer a musculoskeletal injury, such as a strain or sprain, then unless it is serious enough to require urgent medical attention, you should adhere to the RICE – Rest, Ice, Compression and Elevation – approach of treating it, as recommended by sports physiotherapists:

Rest: Take your body weight off the injured area as soon as you can. Rest for 24–48 hours.

Ice: Apply ice to the injured area for 6–10 minutes, every 2–3 hours, using either a specialist ice pack or a bag of frozen peas wrapped in a tea towel to avoid a painful burn.

Compression: Apply an elasticated or other compression bandage to the area to limit the spread of fluids that accumulate as a result of swelling and internal bleeding.

Elevation: Whenever possible, try to keep the injured body part raised and well supported so that the fluids produced by bleeding and swelling drain away. This is particularly important with leg injuries to ensure fluids don't pool at your feet.

Repeat the **RICE** strategy for 28–48 hours before attempting to apply weight to or mobilise the area. If it's still too painful, seek medical advice.

PREGNANCY: Thirty years ago the advice to pregnant women was that a gentle stroll was their physical limit and they should cover no more than a mile a day. Now researchers have

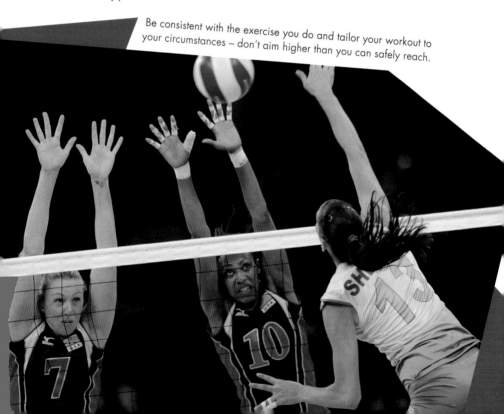

Be consistent with the exercise you do and tailor your workout to your circumstances – don't aim higher than you can safely reach.

confirmed that exercise is not only safe but beneficial for both mother and baby. However, many expectant mothers still put their feet up, with one study of more than 150,000 pregnant women showing that most did not meet the minimum requirement of activity for healthy expectant mothers – 30 minutes of moderate exercise a day. Many wrongly believed that exercise damages an unborn child by starving it of blood and oxygen. In fact, a woman's heart pumps more blood than normal to ensure the foetus is not deprived when she works out. Always seek the advice of your doctor or midwife before exercising in case there are complications with your pregnancy, but non-weight-bearing activities, such as brisk walking, swimming or cycling, are often the best ways to stay active.

CREATE BALANCE: Make sure there is a sense of balance to your lifestyle – don't restrict your exercise to the weekends or cram it into a couple of days. Squeezing your physical activity into two days puts more intense strain on your body and doesn't increase your fitness levels as effectively as less but more consistent activity over the week. Remember to rest. Allow time for your body to recover and adapt to activity, especially if trying something new. Active recovery, like a gentle walk the day after something strenuous, will help you avoid overtraining and injury.

RESPECT YOUR AGE: Exercise has no age barriers and the number of people staying active later in life is higher than ever before. One in 10 Britons aged 55–64 and 5 per cent of over-65s now attend a gym regularly, while many more keep fit by other means. However, if you are returning to exercise after a few years of inactivity, don't just dive in expecting to achieve what you did 10–15 years ago. As you get older, you lose water content from all the body's structures, including cartilage that protects joints. Tissues become weaker and less compliant, which means injuries happen more easily. In short, the older you are, the more important it is that you are well prepared for working out. Listen to your body and modify your exercise to meet your current needs and ability.

Nutrition

Food is fuel for athletes: consume the wrong sort of diet and, like a car engine supplied with the wrong fuel, their bodies will flounder as they struggle to summon up the energy they need to move smoothly and efficiently. Likewise, in order to get the best out of yourself, you need to eat a healthy balanced diet that provides the right type of energy to support your active lifestyle. The trick is not to lose your way in today's healthy-eating maze and to get the essential nutrients you need from foods you enjoy.

Base your meals on carbohydrates with a low Glycaemic Index (GI) rating such as lentils, oats and wholegrain pasta. They release sugars into the body more slowly and evenly leaving you feeling fuller for longer. High GI foods such as cakes, biscuits, white bread and highly processed foods cause blood sugar levels to soar and then crash, sometimes triggering a cycle of hunger, snacking and weight gain.

Include some low-fat protein, such as lean meat, fish and eggs, in your meals. Protein is needed by every cell in the body and plays an important role in muscle recovery after exercise.

Fat gets a bad rap but problems only arise when we eat too much. The current recommendation is to get no more than 35 per cent of your total calorie intake from fat and less than 10 per cent of all calories should be saturated animal fats, such as butter and lard. Trans-fatty acids found in margarines and spreads that contain hydrogenated plant oils should be limited. Choose healthy fats such as those in fish oils, olive oil, avocado and most nuts.

Fresh fruit and vegetables are packed with disease-fighting fibre and antioxidant vitamins. An intake of at least five portions a day –

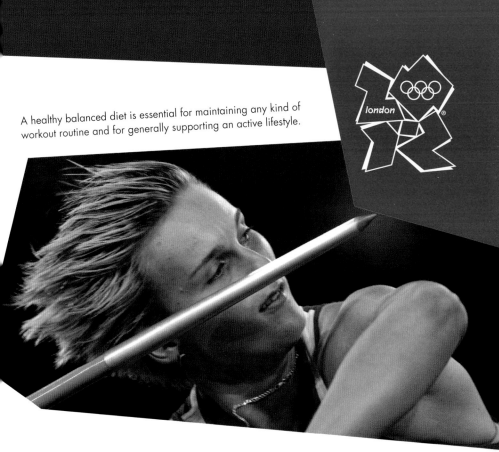

A healthy balanced diet is essential for maintaining any kind of workout routine and for generally supporting an active lifestyle.

one portion of fruit is a slice of melon or two satsumas; a portion of vegetables is equivalent to three tablespoonfuls of carrots and peas – is linked to a lower incidence of cancer, heart disease and other killers. Fresh, frozen, chilled and canned produce all count towards the total. A glass of fruit juice counts as one portion, but you can only count one glass a day as it contains very little fibre. Potatoes don't count towards your five a day because of their high starch content.

Stay in calorie balance if you want to avoid weight gain. All faddy diets, whatever their USP, are ultimately based on this principle. Government guidelines suggest an average female needs 1,940 calories a day to stay healthy, a figure based on a sedentary lifestyle. Although calorie needs vary according to your height, build and genetics, you will need more than that if you are leading an active lifestyle. Most women who follow a fitness programme need to consume around 3,000 calories a day.

FLUID INTAKE

So essential is fluid intake to performance that all of Britain's Olympians undergo sweat analysis tests so that they can accurately pinpoint the amount they need to drink during exercise to avoid dehydration. Maintaining fluid balance in the body is essential at all times, as water is needed for every bodily function. But it is particularly important when you are active. If the average adult loses 1.3–1.8kg of fluid, their athletic performance is seriously impaired. If they lose 3kg, which is possible in hot weather, they are likely to get cramps, nausea and experience a 20–30 per cent drop in endurance capacity.

Drink enough:

No two people have the same sweat rate – it can vary as much among top athletes as the rest of the population. So how much do you need to drink? The average woman needs around 1.8 litres of fluid a day just to stay healthy, but that amount increases if they are active or the weather is warm. During exercise, the majority of people will need to take on board up to 500ml of fluid per hour after the first 45 minutes of intense activity.

Keep a close eye on your fluid intake: stay hydrated, but don't drink too much.

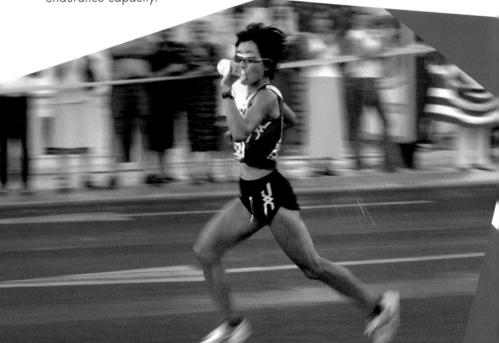

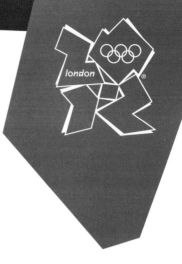

But not too much:

Consuming too much fluid during exercise raises the risk of hyponatremia – or fluid intoxication – a condition that is more prevalent in some endurance sports than dehydration. Caused by depleted levels of sodium and other body salts, it can result in dizziness, vomiting, respiratory problems and fatigue. During intense or prolonged exercise, the kidneys are unable to excrete fluid as efficiently as normal. In extreme cases, water is retained, especially in highly absorbent brain cells, and the pressure causes the body to shut down its primary functions, such as breathing and heart rate. Treatment involves a small volume of highly concentrated salt solution. But hyponatremia can be fatal.

What type of fluid:

It's not only plain water that has the power to rehydrate. Foods such as soups, stews, fruit and vegetables contain high levels of water, and even tea and coffee count towards your daily fluid intake. Athletes often use isotonic sports drinks, containing electrolytes (or body salts) and particles of easily digested carbohydrates that enable the body to absorb fluid more efficiently and also top up levels of glycogen. However, sports drinks are not necessary unless you are undertaking intense or prolonged training programmes lasting one hour or more.

Motivation

For Olympic athletes it may be the pursuit of a medal or a place in a final. For others who exercise it could be the thrill of knowing that their body has been pushed to unknown extremes, or simply the satisfaction of doing something solely for themselves. Whatever it is that motivates you to work out, these unique inspirational factors are crucial to the success of your fitness programme.

Motivation underpins any exercise goal: without it we are almost certainly doomed to give up at the first hurdle. But while some of us have bucket-loads of motivation, others struggle to muster the amount needed to get their trainers on and start moving. So what sets people apart? Sports psychologists say that personality plays a part in determining how naturally self-motivated you are. But just as someone can train to run or cycle faster, so they can work to improve their levels of motivation.

There are two basic motivational forces that influence someone's tendency to keep up – or give up

– fitness workouts. When someone first takes up exercise, it is likely to be 'extrinsic' factors, such as weight loss or the chance of collecting sponsorship money, that drives them to continue. But extrinsic motivation is usually self-limiting – once newcomers achieve their external goals, they are more likely to quit.

Once exercise becomes an enjoyable habit, then intrinsic motivational factors take over. Goals become internalised, so that something like achieving a personal best time, rather than dropping a dress size, becomes the main aim. Intrinsically motivated people are far less likely to quit. Extrinsic motivation will always have

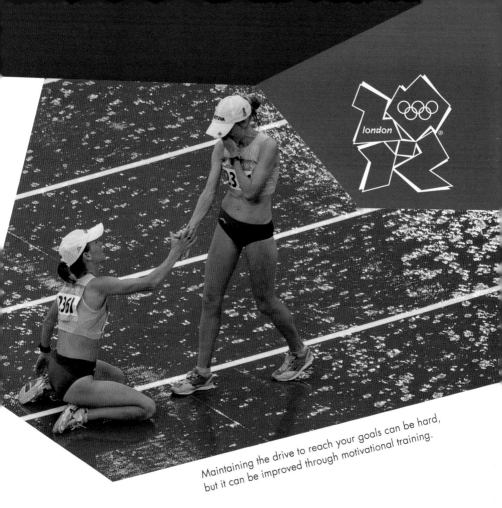

Maintaining the drive to reach your goals can be hard, but it can be improved through motivational training.

its place, but elite athletes know that the psychological route to success lies in enhancing the motivational forces that lie within. Much of the emotional training practised by top athletes can be applied to any fitness programme. Positive thinking and self-talk, emotional conditioning to withstand pre-competition nerves and visualising success are all key to performing well. Setting goals, and realising they are not a constant but evolve and change according to your situation, is also important. People who successfully re-boot their motivation on a regular basis are constantly re-evaluating their fitness aims. And remember that even Olympic athletes have days (or weeks) when motivation flags. Get through these periods, though, and the mental strength that comes with knowing you can pull through is immense.

Eight ways to boost motivation

The road to Olympic glory is pitted with a host of mental and physical barriers. To overcome the setbacks and periods of tedium, sports psychologists have developed a portfolio of techniques to help athletes keep themselves motivated. Some of the same techniques can be used by anyone wanting to give their fitness routine a mental boost:

Keep a training diary: Writing down your goals and achievements in a training diary (see pages 222–223) is a simple but hugely rewarding step. On a day when you are struggling to find motivation to exercise, flicking back through the pages to see how far you have come since you started can be a big enough incentive to get you moving.

Set SMART goals: In sports psychology speak, the acronym SMART stands for Specific, Measurable, Action-oriented, Realistic (but challenging) and Time-sensitive goals. In practical terms, this means setting shorter- and medium-term goals en route to your long-term aim. Setting one long-term goal, such as running a marathon, can be counterproductive for many people, as they get overwhelmed by the scale of the task ahead. Setting the task of first running a 5km, then a 10km race and a half-marathon before you tackle 26.2 miles can help to keep you motivated.

Make some goals public: Want to run a 5km event or compete in a triathlon? Whether you write down your intentions and pin them up on the fridge or tell all your friends what you are doing, it enhances the chance of you sticking to your ultimate aim.

Give yourself personal feedback: Re-evaluate your goals and achievements regularly. If you fail to meet a particular goal, make sure you learn from it so that it becomes a positive experience. It could be that you set an unrealistic goal or that your technique needs adjusting. Remember that trying something, even if it doesn't work, is a step forward in fitness and sport.

Don't get in a workout rut: Make sure you add variety to your programme. Dull and repetitive workouts can backfire – a study at the University of Florida found that doing exactly the same form of exercise over several months greatly increased the chances of someone giving up altogether.

Visualise your success: Visualisation techniques are a staple of any top athlete's portfolio of mental tricks. If you can visualise something in your mind – such as playing the perfect shot in tennis, performing the perfect somersault or cycling up a particularly tough hill – and replay it over and again, then the chances of you successfully doing it are raised considerably.

Use dissociation techniques: At the tough points in a marathon, world record-holder Paula Radcliffe counts to 100 or repeats her daughter's name over and over again. Why? Because she is practising a technique known as dissociation in which you divert attention away from pain and fatigue. If you are struggling through a workout, try counting the number of colours you can see around you or work your way through the alphabet for a chosen category, such as girls' names or sports stars. Before you know it the pain or fatigue (and the workout) will be over.

Reward yourself: For Olympic athletes, rewards come in the form of medals and records. But what about the rest of us? If you have met one of your goals, however small, don't be afraid to reward yourself with a meal out with friends or a new item of clothing. You deserve it.

Troubleshooting

As you push your body through new fitness boundaries, you may find you experience unexpected niggles and unexplained ailments. Don't worry – you are not alone. Workout problems sometimes plague even the fittest, fastest and strongest athletes in the world. Use the troubleshooting guide below to find out what might be wrong.

I always get a side stitch when I exercise. What causes it?

People prone to stitch often have weak core abdominal muscles. During exercise, our internal organs bounce up and down, pulling on the diaphragm muscles. If this tugging occurs when the diaphragm moves upwards – or when we breathe out – the strain is so great it causes a stitch. Sometimes the problem is linked to dehydration. Drinking little and often during exercise should help, as should avoiding a heavy meal within 2–3 hours of exercising.

I have weak ankles that are prone to twisting or spraining. Is there anything I can do to strengthen them?

Balance training using an inexpensive tool called a wobble board – a board attached to half a ball that provides an unstable platform to stand on – is a tool widely used by elite athletes and is among the best means of strengthening ankles. Dutch researchers, reporting in the *British Medical Journal,* found that athletes who practised moves such as standing on one leg and using a wobble board three times a week for eight weeks were 35 per cent less likely to suffer ankle injuries in the following 12 months. Balance training also improves proprioception – your body's sense of muscle awareness and position.

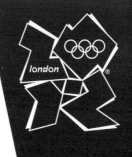

Why do I get headaches when I work out?

Exercise headaches are surprisingly common. If you suffer a pounding head after a workout, the chances are it will be what is known as a 'benign exertional headache'. They can last for up to 24 hours, are usually recurrent, but treatment with non-steroidal, anti-inflammatory drugs can prevent them. Another possibility is the 'effort migraine', which usually happens during exercise and tends to occur in people with a family history of migraines. This can be prevented with a thorough and gradual warm-up before you start. A thumping head is a common symptom of PMS, with a study published in the journal *Neurology* showing that women are twice as likely to report migraine headaches in the two days before their period.

I have a persistent aching in the front of my lower legs. What's the matter?

The likely problem is shin splints, characterised by a dull but considerable pain in the front of the legs and often occurring as a result of doing too much exercise too soon. Shin splints happen when tendons – the tough bands of tissue that connect muscle to bone – or the lining of the shin bone become inflamed after absorbing too much impact during strenuous activity. Sports most likely to produce shin splints include running, or activities such as aerobics in which a lot of jumping is involved. The best way to avoid them is to progress your exercise regime gradually and vary your workout routine to ensure you are getting stronger. Try the gentle stretches in the flexibility section. Swimming can also help.

Exercise seems to increase my bowel movements. Why is this?

Desperately needing the loo is one of the most common reasons for a pit stop during exercise. But what causes the problem that is sometimes dubbed runner's trots (even though it can occur during all types of exercise)? In some people, the combination of increased gut movement and a redirection of blood flow during physical activity results in the release of chemicals that can trigger a bowel movement or diarrhoea. The symptoms seem more common in those who become dehydrated, so taking on enough fluid during long runs can help. But avoid warm drinks like coffee before you start, as they can trigger the problem in some people.

I experience pain in my elbow when I try to lift or hit anything with my arm. What is causing it?

Commonly called 'tennis elbow', this kind of joint pain is usually caused by repeated contractions of muscles connected to the elbow of your hitting arm in tennis and other sports, such as golf and badminton, although it can also be triggered by doing too much housework or weight training. As you perform these activities, shock forces reverberate up the forearm into the elbow, causing the pain. The more you use the joint, the worse it can get. Wrist-strengthening exercises, such as repeatedly squeezing a tennis ball, can help to strengthen the forearms. If you play racket sports, improve your technique through coaching and make sure your racket grip is the right size.

I get recurrent pain in my knees. What might be causing it?

Active women are up to eight times more likely to suffer knee problems than sporty men, partly because the wider angle of their hips puts added stress on the knees when working out, but also because hormones, such as oestrogen, weaken ligaments at different phases of the menstrual cycle, leaving them prone to twisting or straining. Researchers at the University of Calgary found that the timing of hormone-induced laxity – or flexibility – of joints varies among women, with most experiencing some pain or discomfort around ovulation, but others displaying a greater predisposition to knee and joint problems at the very start or end of their cycle. Adjust your training programme to avoid high-impact workouts if your knees ache at certain times of the month. Try swimming or cycling instead.

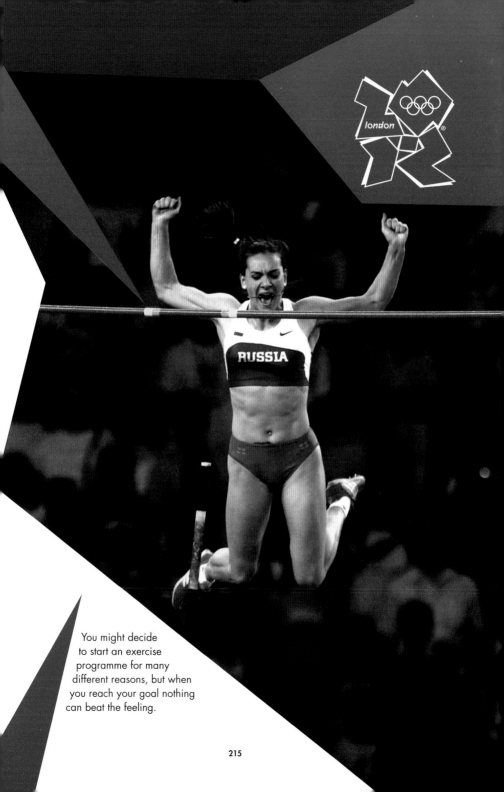

You might decide
to start an exercise
programme for many
different reasons, but when
you reach your goal nothing
can beat the feeling.

215

Glossary

Aerobic capacity: Maximal oxygen uptake (or VO_2 Max).

Aerobic exercise: Activity in which the body is able to supply adequate oxygen to the working muscles for a sustained period of time.

Aerobic fitness: The body's ability to take in and use oxygen during prolonged activity.

Anaerobic exercise: Short bursts of 'all-out' activities, such as sprinting or weightlifting, which do not rely on the muscles being supplied with oxygen.

Antioxidants: The vitamins A, C and E and various minerals that protect the body by preventing oxidation, a process that produces damaging free radical substances.

Biomechanics: The study of internal and external forces of the body and of how those forces influence movement.

Body composition: The unique breakdown of your body make-up, including percentages of lean muscle, bone and water content.

Bone density: The thickness and solid structure of the bones within the body.

Calorie: Unit of energy.

Cardiovascular training/fitness: Physical activity that strengthens the heart and blood vessels.

Chronic injury/pain: An injury or problem that develops and continues over a period of months or years.

Cool-down: Post-exercise activity designed to return the body to its resting state.

Core stability: Strength in the muscles of the trunk that work to stabilise the body and spine.

Coronary Heart Disease (CHD): Diseases of the heart muscle and the blood vessels that supply it with oxygen.

Cross-training: Varying your fitness workouts and training to challenge different muscles and energy systems.

Dehydration: Excessive fluid loss through sweat, urination, diarrhoea or sickness.

Delayed Onset Muscle Soreness (DOMS): Post-exercise stiffness and soreness that occur 24–48 hours after a workout.

Dumbbell: Small, hand-held weight with detachable discs or fixed weights at each end.

Dynamic stretching: Flexibility exercises involving movement. **Energy expenditure:** The amount of energy used in activity, measured in kilocalories.

Extension: Moving a body part from a bent to a straight position, as in leg extension.

Flexibility: The range of movement in a joint or group of joints.

Flexion: The movement of a body part from straight to bent.

Free radical: Substance produced in the body or from smoke or pollutants that can damage cells and the body's DNA.

Gluteals: Term used to describe the gluteus maximus, medius and minimus muscles in the hips and buttocks.

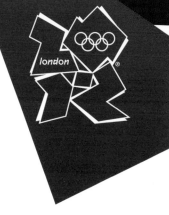

Glycemic Index (GI): A classification system for a food's ability to raise blood sugar levels.

Glycogen: The stored form of carbohydrate energy (glucose) in the muscles and liver.

Heart rate: A measurement of the work done by the heart, normally expressed as the number of beats per minute (bpm).

Hypertension: High blood pressure.

Interval training: Intense bursts of exercise followed by periods of recovery.

Isotonic drink: A fluid containing particles of carbohydrates at the same concentration as the body's own fluid.

Lactic acid: A waste product caused by anaerobic training of the muscles, a build-up of which leads to fatigue.

Lean body mass: Total levels of muscle tissue in the body.

Ligaments: Tissue that connects bone to bone.

Muscle: Tissue consisting of fibres organised into bands or bundles that contract to trigger movement.

Musculoskeletal: Referring to muscles and bones.

Oestrogen: A principal female hormone.

Overload principle: Applying a greater load than normal to a muscle to increase its strength.

Overtraining: High levels of exercise that are detrimental to health and fitness.

Pedometer: A device that counts steps taken when walking or running.

Power: Force applied at speed.

Proprioception: Muscle awareness and stability.

Rate of Perceived Exertion (RPE): A self-reported rating of how hard you are working.

Reps: Abbreviation for repetitions, the number of times an exercise is performed.

Resistance training: Training methods, often using weights, to increase the body's strength, power and muscular endurance.

RICE: Rest, Ice, Compression and Elevation – a strategy for treating injuries.

Set: A group of repetitions.

Stamina: Endurance levels or aerobic fitness.

Static stretch: A move that is held in the stretched position for several seconds.

Strength training: The use of resistance weight training to build maximum muscle force.

Tendon: A band of fibrous tissue that connects muscle to bone.

VO_2 Max: The maximum amount of oxygen a person can utilise per minute of work.

Warm-up: Light-gradual exercises performed to get the body ready for exercise.

What next?

A stronger, fitter body can provide you with the confidence and self-belief to aim higher with your physical activity goals. If you are inspired to raise your goals, why not try getting involved in an Olympic sport? Many of the governing bodies listed below organise entry-level beginner schemes to encourage newcomers to get involved – whatever their age – or join a club where you will get expert coaching and advice.

Archery
   Archery GB: archerygb.org
   01952 677 888
Athletics
   UK Athletics: uka.org.uk
   0121 713 8400
Badminton
   Badminton England:
   badmintonengland.co.uk
   0190 826 8400
   Badminton Scotland:
   badmintonscotland.org
   0141 445 1218
   Badminton Union of Ireland:
   sportni.org; 0289 038 1222
   Welsh Badminton:
   welshbadminton.net
   0845 045 4301
Basketball
   England Basketball:
   englandbasketball.co.uk
   0114 284 1060
   Basketball Northern Ireland
   basketballni.com; 0289 038 3817

   Basketball Scotland
   basketball-scotland.com
   0131 317 7260
   Welsh Basketball
   basketballwales.com
Boxing
   Amateur Boxing Association of England abae.org.uk; 0114 223 5654
   GB Boxing: gbboxing.org.uk;
   0114 223 5692
Canoeing: Slalom and Sprint
   British Canoe Union: bcu.org.uk
   0845 370 9500 or 0300 011 9500
Track, Road, Mountain Bike and BMX Cycling
   British Cycling: britishcycling.org.uk
   0161 274 2000
Equestrian
   British Equestrian Federation:
   bef.co.uk; 0247 669 8871
Fencing
   British Fencing: britishfencing.com
   020 8742 3032
Football
   The Football Association: thefa.com
   0844 980 8200

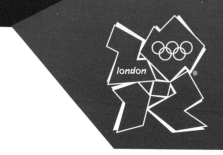

The Football Association of Wales:
faw.org.uk; 0292 043 5830
The Irish Football Association
irishfa.com; 0289 066 9458 *The
Scottish Football Association:*
scottishfa.co.uk; 0141 616 6000
Gymnastics
British Gymnastics:
british-gymnastics.org
0845 1297129
Handball
British Handball Association:
britishhandball.com; 01233 878099
Hockey
Great Britain Hockey
greatbritainhockey.co.uk;
01628 897 509
England Hockey:
englandhockey.co.uk; 0162 889 7500
Ireland Hockey - Ulster Branch
www.ulsterhockey.com; 028 9076 5766
Scottish Hockey:
Scottish-hockey.co.uk; 0131 453 9070
Welsh Hockey Union:
welsh-hockey.co.uk; 0292 078 0730
Judo
British Judo Association:
britishjudo.org.uk 01509 631670
Modern Pentathlon
British Pentathlon: pentathlongb.org
0122 538 6808
Rowing
British Rowing: britishrowing.org
0208 237 6700
Sailing
Royal Yachting Association:
rya.org.uk; 0238 060 4100
Shooting
British Shooting:
britishshooting.org.uk; 01483 486 948

**Swimming, Synchronised Swimming,
Diving and Water Polo**
British Swimming: swimming.org/
britishswimming; 0150 961 8700
Table Tennis
British Table Tennis Association;
0146 267 1191
English Table Tennis Association:
englishtabletennis.org.uk
0142 445 6217
Table Tennis Association of Wales:
ttaw.co.uk
Table Tennis Scotland:
tabletennisscotland.com
0131 317 8077
Irish Table Tennis – Ulster Province
irishtabletennis.com 00 353 1 6251135
Taekwondo
British Taekwondo Control Board:
britishtaekwondo.org.uk
0207 701 3764
Tennis
Lawn Tennis Association:
lta.org.uk; 0208 487 7000
Triathlon
British Triathlon Federation:
britishtriathlon.org; 01509 226161
Volleyball
British Volleyball:
britishvolleyball.org; 0114 223 5730
Weightlifting
British Weightlifting Association:
bwla.co.uk; 0113 812 7098
Wrestling
British Wrestling:
britishwrestling.org; 0124 623 6443

Index

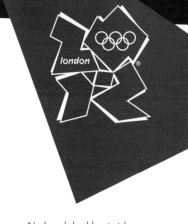

Training diary

A training diary is perhaps the most important motivational tool to back up your workouts.

Here is a sample layout of a training diary page which you can photocopy for your own use. Below are some suggestions about what it might be useful to include:

1. Sleep record: Keeping track of the hours of sleep you get can help you to assess if your sleeping patterns are affecting your performance.
2. Personal goals: Set specific goals for each session. This helps to focus the mind and means you are much more likely to achieve the results you desire.
3. Weight: Recording your weight once a week (but no more) can help to make sure your programme is on track if weight loss is one of your goals.
4. How it felt: Write down anything that might make future workouts go more smoothly. Did you feel one exercise was harder than the others? This information can be valuable in the weeks ahead.
5. Heart rate: Keeping a record of your resting heart rate (taken in the morning) is helpful to make sure things are remaining on an even keel.

Date/Time	Description of acti

ration	Motivational target	Additional notes

Keep going

Picture credits

The publishers would like to thank the following sources for their kind permission to reproduce the pictures in this book.

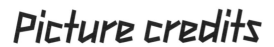

All the dedication paid off for Australian sprinter Cathy Freeman, who won the 400 metres at the 2000 Olympic Games in Sydney.